Pharmacy Registration
Assessment Questions 2

Pharmacy Registration Assessment Questions 2

Nadia Bukhari (Series Managing Editor)

BPharm, PG Dip Pharm Prac, PG Dip T&L in Higher Ed, MRPharmS, FHEA
Clinical Lecturer, Pre-Registration Co-ordinator & MPharm Student Support Manager, UCL School of Pharmacy

Oksana Pyzik (Assistant Editor)

MPharm, MRPharmS
Senior Teaching Fellow at the UCL School of Pharmacy in the Department of Practice and Policy

Ryan Hamilton (Contributor)

PhD, PGCert(Clinical Pharmacy), MFRPSI, MPharm(Hons), AMRSC, AFHEA
Specialist Pharmacist in Antimicrobials & Acute Medicine, University Hospitals of Leicester NHS Trust and active member of the UK Clinical Pharmacy Association's infection network

Simon Harris (Contributor)

MPharm, MRPharmS
Education and Training Lead at Green Light Campus and Pre-Reg Training Manager for Green Light Pharmacy

Harshar Parmar (Contributor)

MPharm, MRPharmS
Senior Lecturer in Pharmacy Practice, University of Manchester, practising community pharmacist

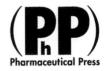

Pharmaceutical Press

Published by the Pharmaceutical Press
66–68 East Smithfield, London E1W 1AW, UK

© Pharmaceutical Press 2018

(**PP**) is a trade mark of Pharmaceutical Press

Pharmaceutical Press is the publishing division of the Royal Pharmaceutical Society

First published 2018

Reprinted 2019

Typeset by SPi Global, Chennai, India
Printed in Great Britain by Hobbs the Printers, Totton, Hampshire

ISBN 978 0 85711 326 9 (print)
ISBN 978 0 85711 325 2 (mobi)
ISBN 978 0 85711 327 6 (epdf)
ISBN 978 0 85711 328 3 (ePub)

A catalogue record for this book is available from the British Library

Disclaimer
The views expressed in this book are solely those of the author and do not necessarily reflect the views or policies of the Royal Pharmaceutical Society. This book does NOT guarantee success in the registration exam but can be used as an aid for revision.

To all the trainee pharmacists: dream big, aim high; always believe in yourselves.

Nadia Bukhari 2018

Contents

Preface

After the overwhelming success of our first four volumes of *Registration Exam Questions*, a decision was made to launch a new series named *Pharmacy Registration Assessment Questions* (PRAQ). In this new series we hope to incorporate questions that are aligned to the new GPhC Framework and incorporate a similar style of questions to what has recently been announced by the GPhC for the Registration Assessment.

Both editions of volume 1 have been well received, hence encouraging the writing of a new volume.

Volume 2 of PRAQ is a bank of just under 500 questions, which are similar to the style of the registration examination. The majority of the questions are based on law and ethics, and clinical pharmacy and therapeutic aspects of the registration examination syllabus, as well as pharmaceutical calculations.

After completing 4 years of study and graduating with a Master of Pharmacy (MPharm) degree, graduates are required to undertake training as a pre-registration pharmacist before they can sit the registration examination.

Pre-registration training is the period of employment on which graduates must embark and effectively complete before they can register as a pharmacist in the UK. In most cases it is a 1-year period after the pharmacy degree; for sandwich course students it is integrated within the undergraduate programme.

On successfully passing the registration examination, pharmacy graduates can register as a pharmacist in the UK.

The registration examination harmonises the testing of skills in practice during the pre-registration year. It tests:

- knowledge
- the application of knowledge
- calculation
- time management
- managing stress
- comprehension

- recall
- interpretation
- evaluation.

There are two examination papers: Paper 1 (calculations paper with extracts) and Paper 2 (closed book paper with extracts). Questions are based on practice-based situations and are designed to test the thinking and knowledge that lie behind any action.

EXAMINATION FORMAT

The registration examination consists of two papers:

1   Paper 1: calculations with extracts

- free text answers; calculators can be used (only models approved by GPhC)
- 40 calculations in 120 minutes (2 hours)
- extracts from reference sources provided for questions that require additional information.

2   Paper 2: closed book with extracts

- multiple-choice question (MCQ) paper with extracts from reference sources provided
- 120 questions in 150 minutes (2.5 hours).

Two types of MCQs are used:

- 90 single best answer questions
- 30 extended matching questions.

The registration examination is crucial for pharmacy graduates wishing to register in the UK.

Due to student demand, *Pharmacy Registration Assessment Questions* will be an annual publication with brand-new questions for students to attempt. We hope to include questions on most aspects of the examination and will take any changes made by the GPhC into consideration.

Preparation is the key. This book cannot guarantee that you will pass the registration assessment; however, it can help you to identify your learning needs and practice questions with themes and elements from within the GPhC framework questions. And, as they say, 'practice makes perfect'.

This book is written with the most current *BNF* at the time of writing. Please use the most current *BNF* and reference sources when using this book.

Good luck with the preparation and the assessment.

Nadia Bukhari
January 2018

Acknowledgements

The editor wishes to acknowledge the support from colleagues at the UCL School of Pharmacy.

Thank you to all four contributors: Oksana Pyzik, Simon Harris, Harsha Parmar and Ryan Hamilton.

Nadia Bukhari would like to express thanks to the editors at Pharmaceutical Press for their support and patience in the writing of this book, and especially to Mark Pollard for his guidance.

About the authors

Nadia Bukhari BPharm, PG Dip Pharm Prac, PG Dip T&L in Higher Ed, MRPharmS, FHEA

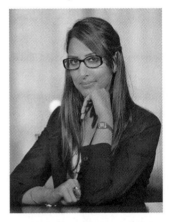

Nadia Bukhari is the Chair of the RPS Pre-registration Conferences. She developed the extremely popular and over-subscribed conference, when it first started in 2012. Nadia graduated from the School of Pharmacy, University of London in 1999. After qualifying, she worked as a pharmacy manager at Westbury Chemist, Streatham for a year, after which she moved on to work for Bart's and the London NHS Trust as a clinical pharmacist in surgery. It was at this time that Nadia developed an interest in teaching, because part of her role involved the responsibility of being a teacher practitioner for the School of Pharmacy, University of London. Two and a half years later, she commenced working for the School of Pharmacy, University of London as the pre-registration coordinator and the academic facilitator. This position involved teaching therapeutics to Master of Pharmacy students and assisting the director of undergraduate studies.

While teaching undergraduate students, Nadia completed her Post Graduate Diploma in Pharmacy Practice and her Post Graduate Diploma in Teaching in Higher Education. She then took on the role of the Master of Pharmacy Programme Manager, which involved the management of the undergraduate degree as well as being the pre-registration coordinator for the university.

Since the merger with UCL, Nadia has now taken on the role of Senior Teaching Fellow in Pharmacy Practice and is the pre-registration coordinator and alumni coordinator for the university. She is also a Fellow of the Higher Education Academy and is the module lead for the final year pharmacy practice course.

Taking her research interest further, Nadia is currently in the fifth year of her PhD, which she is doing on a part-time basis. Her research area is 'leadership in pharmacy'.

Nadia's interest in writing emerged in her first year of working in academia. Thirteen years on, Nadia has authored six titles with the Pharmaceutical Press. She is currently writing her eighth title, which is due to be published in February 2018.

Nadia is a Fellow of the Royal Pharmaceutical Society, in recognition of her distinction in the profession of pharmacy and is an elected Board member for the English Pharmacy Board.

Dr Ryan Hamilton PhD, PGCert(Clinical Pharmacy), MFRPSI, MPharm (Hons), AMRSC, AFHEA

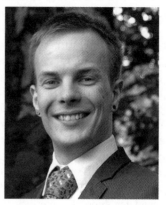

Ryan Hamilton is a specialist pharmacist at the University Hospitals of Leicester NHS Trust, where he works within the fields of antimicrobials and acute medicine.

Ryan studied pharmacy at Liverpool John Moore's University, to which he returned after completing his preregistration training at King's College Hospital, London, to undertake a PhD in pharmaceutical sciences. His research investigates the interaction of antimicrobial agents with clay minerals and the development of candidate materials for the treatment of infected wounds.

Throughout his career Ryan has supported pharmacy students and pre-registration pharmacists. As President of the British Pharmaceutical Students' Association, he developed guidance for students and trainees, and worked closely with the GPhC to ensure trainees were fairly represented. Ryan now acts as an ambassador for the BPSA and sits on the RPS's Education Forum where he represents trainees and foundation year pharmacists.

Harsha Parmar MPharm, MRPharmS

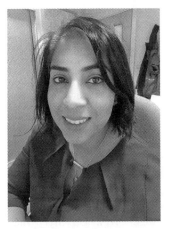

Harsha Parmar is a Senior Lecturer in Pharmacy Practice at the University of Manchester and practising community pharmacist. Harsha's teaching is informed through both a formal postgraduate qualification in teaching, learning and assessment, and her ongoing active practice as a pharmacist. Her teaching portfolio involves extensive experience in the curriculum design and delivery of public health, pharmacy law and ethics, dispensing, minor ailments, pharmaceutical care, disease management and advanced consultation skills. She has completed a Masters in Philosophy focusing on preparedness for practice of pharmacy students. Harsha is a Senior Fellow of the Higher education academy, which recognises her work in the leadership of teaching, learning and assessment in the field of pharmacy education.

Oksana Pyzik MPharm, MRPharmS

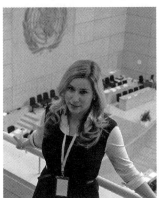

Oksana Pyzik is a Senior Teaching Fellow and Global Engagement Coordinator at University College London (UCL) School of Pharmacy. In addition to her role in education, Oksana is also a Global Health Advisor and Board Trustee of the Commonwealth Pharmacists Association. Oksana first started her career as a pharmacist in the primary care setting delivering public health interventions to marginalised patient groups in underserved communities across London. It was this early experience in practice that motivated her to conduct public health research at the International Pharmaceutical Federation (FIP) before moving into the academic sector full time in 2013. She went on to earn her Post Graduate Diploma in Teaching and Learning in Higher Professional Education at the Institute of Education in 2015 and is now a Fellow of the UK Higher Education Academy. Oksana is extensively involved with the Royal Pharmaceutical Society (RPS) Preregistration Conferences in both the development of teaching material and the delivery of training sessions. She also remains active in community pharmacy setting, serving as the 'Preregistration and Academic Lead' for the Central London Local Practice Forum (LPF) where she acts as a link between community pharmacy and academia in this role.

Simon Harris MPharm, MRPharmS

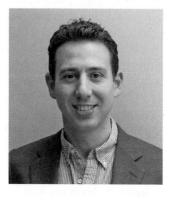

Simon Harris graduated from the University of Strathclyde, Glasgow in 2002. After spending his pre-registration year working in the hospital sector, he switched to community pharmacy on registration. Simon is now the Education and Training Lead at Green Light Campus and Pre-Reg Training Manager for Green Light Pharmacy, where he runs the highly regarded Green Light Pre-Registration Study Day Programme, and develops and delivers training at monthly study days to pre-registration trainees from across England (more info at www.greenlightpharmacy.com). Simon is also an Honorary Lecturer at UCL School of Pharmacy, where he is part of the pharmacy practice team, as well as a London Events Tutor with CPPE, where he facilitates workshops on a wide variety of clinical topics in central and north London.

Abbreviations

ACBS	Advisory Committee on Borderline Substances
ACE	angiotensin-converting enzyme
ACEI	angiotensin-converting enzyme inhibitor
ACS	acute coronary syndrome
AF	atrial fibrillation
ALT DIE	alternate days
AV	arteriovenous
BD	twice daily
BMI	body mass index
BNF	*British National Formulary*
BNFC	*British National Formulary for Children*
BP	blood pressure
BPSA	British Pharmaceutical Students' Association
BSA	body surface area
BTS	British Thoracic Society
CCF	congestive/chronic cardiac failure
CD	controlled drug
CDC	US Centers for Disease Control and Prevention
CE	*conformité européenne*
CFC	chlorofluorocarbon
CHM	Commission on Human Medicines
CHMP	Committee for Medicinal Products for Human Use
CI	confidence interval or cumulative incidence
CKS	Clinical Knowledge Summaries
COX	cyclooxygenase
COPD	chronic obstructive pulmonary disease
CPD	continuing professional development
CPPE	Centre for Pharmacy Postgraduate Education
CrCl	creatinine clearance (mL/min)
CSM	Committee on Safety of Medicines
CYT	cytochrome
DigCl	digoxin clearance (L/h)

DMARD	disease-modifying antirheumatic drug
DNG	discount not given
DPF	*Dental Practitioners' Formulary*
DPI	dry-powder inhaler
EC	enteric-coated
ECG	electrocardiogram
EEA	European Economic Area
eGFR	estimated glomerular filtration rate
EHC	emergency hormonal contraception
F1	Foundation Year 1
FEV_1	forced expiratory volume in 1 second
GP	general practitioner
GP6D	glucose-6-phosphate dehydrogenase
GPhC	General Pharmaceutical Council
GSL	general sales list
GTN	glyceryl trinitrate
HbA1c	glycated haemoglobin
HDU	high dependency unit
HIV	human immunodeficiency virus
HR	heart rate
HRT	hormone replacement therapy
IBS	irritable bowel syndrome
IBW	ideal body weight
IDA	industrial denatured alcohol
IM	intramuscular
INR	international normalised ratio
IV	intravenous
IUD	intrauterine device
MAOI	monoamine oxidase inhibitor
MD	maximum single dose
MDD	maximum daily dose
MDI	metered-dose inhaler
MDU	to be used as directed
MEP	*Medicines, Ethics and Practice* guide
MHRA	Medicines and Healthcare products Regulatory Agency
MMR	measles, mumps and rubella
MR, m/r	modified release
MRSA	meticillin-resistant *Staphylococcus aureus*
MUPS	multiple-unit pellet system
MUR	Medicines Use Review
NHS	National Health Service

NICE	National Institute for Health and Care Excellence
NMS	New Medicines Service
NRLS	National Reporting and Learning System
NSAIDs	non-steroidal anti-inflammatory drugs
OC	oral contraceptive
OD	*omni die* (every day)
OM	*omni mane* (every morning)
ON	*omni nocte* (every night)
OP	original pack
OPAT	outpatient parenteral antibacterial therapy
ORT	oral rehydration therapy
OTC	over-the-counter
P	pharmacy
PAGB	Proprietary Association of Great Britain
PCT	primary care trust
PHE	Public Health England
PIL	patient information leaflet
pMDI	pressurised metered-dose inhaler
PMR	patient medical record
POM	prescription-only medicine
POM-V	prescription-only medicine – veterinarian
POM-VPS	prescription-only medicine – veterinarian, pharmacist, suitably qualified person
PPIs	proton pump inhibitors
PRN	when required
PSA	prostate-specific antigen
PSNC	Pharmaceutical Services Negotiating Committee
QDS	*quarter die sumendum* (to be taken four times daily)
RCT	randomised controlled trial
RE	right eye
RPS	Royal Pharmaceutical Society (formerly RPSGB)
SARSS	Suspected Adverse Reaction Surveillance Scheme
SCRIPT	Standard Computerised Revalidation Instrument for Prescribing and Therapeutics
SeCr	serum creatinine
SGLT2	sodium (Na^+)/glucose co-transporter 2
SHO	senior house officer
SIGN	Scottish Intercollegiate Guidelines Network
SLS	selected list scheme
SOP	standard operating procedure
SPC	summary of product characteristics

SSRI	selective serotonin reuptake inhibitor
ST	an isoelectric line after the QRS complex of an ECG
STAT	immediately
TCA	tricyclic antidepressant
TDS	three times a day
TIA	transient ischaemic attack
TPN	total parenteral nutrition
TSDA	trade-specific denatured alcohol
U&E	urea and electrolyte count
UTI	urinary tract infection
VITAL	Virtual Interactive Teaching And Learning
WHO	World Health Organization

How to use this book

The book is divided into three main sections: Single best answer questions, Extended matching questions and Calculation questions.

SINGLE BEST ANSWER QUESTIONS (SBAs)

Each of the questions or statements in this section is followed by five suggested answers. Select the best answer in each situation.

For example:
A patient on your ward has been admitted with a gastric ulcer, which is currently being treated. She has a history of arthritis and cardiac problems. Which of her drugs is most likely to have caused the gastric ulcer?

- ☐ A   paracetamol
- ☐ B   naproxen
- ☐ C   furosemide
- ☐ D   propranolol
- ☐ E   codeine phosphate

EXTENDED MATCHING QUESTIONS (EMQs)

Extended matching questions consist of lettered options followed by a list of numbered problems/questions. For each numbered problem/question, select the one lettered option that most closely answers the question. You can use the lettered options once, more than once or not at all.

For example:
Antidepressants

- A   amitriptyline
- B   citalopram
- C   duloxetine
- D   flupentixol

E   mirtazapine
F   moclobemide
G   St John's wort
H   venlafaxine

For questions 1–4
For the patients described, select the single most likely antidepressant from the list above. Each option may be used once, more than once or not at all.

1   Miss K is a 32-year-old woman on your ward who has a long-standing history of depression related to her chronic illness. She has tried antidepressants in the past but stopped them when she felt better. The medical team tell you that she returns to hospital periodically with relapsed symptoms because she stops taking her medicines. They want to treat her depression but the agent they suggest would not be suitable for Miss K, considering her non-adherence.

2   One of the new GPs in the surgery across the road calls you for some advice. He has a patient with him, Mr B, who is 28 years old and has agreed to try an antidepressant medicine. Mr B is otherwise fit and healthy, but the GP would like your advice on what to prescribe for this new diagnosis of moderate depression.

3   Three months later you get another call from the GP about Mr B, who has not responded well to the initial antidepressants and may be experiencing a number of side-effects. They want to switch him on to a different agent quickly, if not immediately. You inform the GP that one of the drugs he asked about cannot be started immediately.

4   Mrs C has just been admitted on to your emergency admissions unit after being referred directly from her GP, whom she went to see about her headache. On admission she also complains of palpitations and her BP is 205/100 mmHg. On taking her history you note she is Japanese and still eats a traditional diet, leading you to suspect her antidepressant medicine may have precipitated this condition.

CALCULATION QUESTIONS

These are free text pharmaceutical calculations. The use of calculators is permitted when tackling these questions. The GPhC will provide candidates with calculators for the purpose of the assessment.

For example:

Mrs D is a 75-year-old woman who has just been admitted to your respiratory ward with an exacerbation of asthma. On admission she was weighed at 97 kg and states her height as 5 feet 3 inches. When taking her history you find she quit smoking 10 years ago and is on the following medicines:

> Fostair 100/6 two puffs BD
> Budesonide 4 mg PO OM
> *Phyllocontin Continus* (aminophylline) 225-mg tablets, two tablets BD MDU
> Salbutamol 2.5 mg nebulised QDS PRN
> Salbutamol 100 mcg CFC-free inhaler 2–6 puffs QDS PRN via an aerochamber (blue)

How much aminophylline should Mrs D receive over the next 24 hours? Give your answer to the nearest whole number.

> The purpose of the registration assessment is to test a candidate's ability to apply the knowledge they have learnt over the past 5 years of their education and training.
>
> Testing someone's ability to locate information efficiently in the *BNF* should be tested during their pre-registration training year and in their undergraduate training.
>
> Therefore, all questions are closed book, with extracts of reference sources provided to candidates.

Answers to the questions are at the end of the book. Brief explanations or a suitable reference for sourcing the answer are given, to aid understanding and to facilitate learning.

Important: this text refers to the current edition of the *BNF* when text was written. Please always consult the LATEST version for the most up-to-date information.

Single best answer questions

Ryan Hamilton

1   Mr Y is a 51-year-old man who has recently had a jejunostomy formed in hospital. He is complaining of increased stoma output and irritation around the stoma site, which his medical team believes is being exacerbated by gastric acid.
Which of the following medicines would be the best first line choice for Mr Y?

    □ A   co-magaldrox
    □ B   *Gaviscon Advance*
    □ C   lansoprazole
    □ D   ranitidine
    □ E   simethicone

2   Mrs D is well known to your pharmacy and has a history of angina, for which she is taking a number of medicines. She presents to your pharmacy with a prescription for isosorbide mononitrate MR 60 mg twice daily. You look at her PMR and see that she was previously prescribed isosorbide mononitrate MR 40 mg twice daily, which she confirms wasn't controlling her symptoms.
What is the best course of action for this patient?

    □ A   Advise Mrs D to stop taking this medicine and supply her with a GTN spray in case of further chest pain
    □ B   Dispense the prescription and tell her to take one dose in the morning and the second dose at lunchtime

☐ **C**   Dispense the prescription but tell the patient to take both doses together rather than splitting them

☐ **D**   Dispense the prescription and tell her to take each dose 12 hours apart

☐ **E**   Discuss the medicine with her GP as it needs to be reviewed

3   Mr W is a 34-year-old man who has been admitted to your acute medical unit with severe leg pain and swelling, which is diagnosed as being a DVT. Whilst undertaking a history for Mr W, you find that he does not take any other medicines and travels abroad for work for prolonged periods.
Which of the following would be the most appropriate treatment option for Mr W?

☐ **A**   aspirin tablets 75 mg OD
☐ **B**   clopidogrel tablets 75 mg OD
☐ **C**   dalteparin injection 15 000 units OD
☐ **D**   rivaroxaban tablets 15 mg BD for 21 days then 20 mg OD
☐ **E**   warfarin tablets 10 mg OD for 2 days, then 5 mg OD for 1 day then as per INR

4   Miss F has just been prescribed a *Duaklir Genuair* 340/12 mcg per dose inhaler for her uncontrolled COPD. She has never used this type of inhaler before so you decide to counsel her on how to use the device. Which of the following instructions is the most appropriate?
You may use the product information leaflet for this product to help you: http://www.medicines.org.uk/emc/PIL.29638.latest.pdf

☐ **A**   Press and release the orange button. Put the inhaler to your mouth. Exhale fully. Then breathe in strongly and deeply

☐ **B**   Press and release the orange button. Exhale fully. Put the inhaler to your mouth. Then breathe in strongly and deeply

☐ **C**   Press the orange button and hold down. Put the inhaler to your mouth. Exhale fully. Then breathe in strongly and deeply. Release the orange button

☐ **D**   Press the orange button and hold down. Exhale fully. Put the inhaler to your mouth. Then breathe in strongly and deeply. Release the orange button

☐ **E**   Shake the inhaler before use. Press and release the orange button. Exhale fully. Put the inhaler to your mouth. Then breathe in strongly and deeply

5   Billy, a 6-year-old boy, has recently been diagnosed with asthma for which his GP has prescribed a beclometasone dipropionate pMDI inhaler, a salbutamol pMDI inhaler and a *Volumatic* spacer. Which of the following is the best advice to give Billy regarding the initial use of salbutamol in acute exacerbations of asthma?

☐ A   Inhale two puffs directly from the inhaler, which can be repeated every 6 hours

☐ B   Inhale two puffs directly from the inhaler, which can be repeated every 10 minutes

☐ C   Inhale one puff using the spacer. This can be repeated once more

☐ D   Inhale one puff using the spacer. This can be repeated every 10 minutes

☐ E   Inhale two to ten puffs, each inhaled separately, using the spacer. This can be repeated every 10 minutes

6   Mrs U has severe depression and is taking moclobemide 300 mg daily, which she has been stable on for around 5 months. She has been admitted to your acute trauma unit with a broken rib due to a fall whilst out shopping. Which of the following analgesia options would be the LEAST appropriate to prescribe for Mrs U?

☐ A   buprenorphine 5 mcg/h patch, one patch every 7 days

☐ B   codeine tablets 30 mg QDS

☐ C   morphine sulfate oral solution, 5–10 mg every 6 hours

☐ D   naproxen tablets 250 mg BD

☐ E   tramadol capsules 100 mg QDS

7   Mr J has been admitted to your urgent care centre with reddening of the skin on his arm after scratching it a few days ago. The doctors believe this is a case of mild cellulitis and prescribe a 5-day course of fusidic acid cream. Assuming that he has no known allergies, what would be the best course of action in this scenario?

☐ A   Dispense the prescription with appropriate counselling

☐ B   Speak to the prescriber and suggest prescribing flucloxacillin orally instead

☐ C   Speak to the prescriber and suggest prescribing flucloxacillin orally alongside the fusidic acid

    ☐ **D** Speak to the prescriber and suggest prescribing vancomycin orally instead

    ☐ **E** Speak to the prescriber and suggest prescribing vancomycin intravenously instead

8   Miss B is a 24-year-old woman who has been admitted to your emergency department with confusion, headache, vomiting and photophobia. After assessment and visual examination of her CSF the medical team make a diagnosis of suspected meningitis. As Miss B has a history of vomiting when taking amoxicillin capsules, the consultant would like to prescribe meropenem.

What advice do you give regarding prescribing this medicine?

You may use the SPC for meropenem to help you: http://www.medicines.org.uk/emc/medicine/24151

    ☐ **A** Prescribe meropenem 500 mg every 8 hours
    ☐ **B** Prescribe meropenem 500 mg every 6 hours
    ☐ **C** Prescribe meropenem 1000 mg every 8 hours
    ☐ **D** Prescribe meropenem 2000 mg every 8 hours
    ☐ **E** Meropenem should not be prescribed as it is also a beta-lactam agent

9   Mrs E is a 47-year-old woman who presents to your pharmacy with a prescription for clotrimazole pessaries as the cream has not worked. She has had recurrent episodes of vaginal thrush and is fed up, but having asked questions about personal hygiene and lifestyle there are no obvious identifiable causes. Whilst reviewing her PMR you note she is on a number of other medicines.

Which of these may be causing her recurrent thrush?

    ☐ **A** amlodipine
    ☐ **B** dapagliflozin
    ☐ **C** metformin
    ☐ **D** ramipril
    ☐ **E** none of the above

10   Mrs F has been taking carbimazole 15 mg OD for the past 3 months pending follow-up from her endocrine team. Today she presents to your pharmacy complaining of a fever and sore throat.

Which of the following is the most appropriate course of action?

- [ ] **A** Offer to supply a simple cough syrup
- [ ] **B** Offer to supply throat lozenges
- [ ] **C** Do not make a supply. Advise the patient that the complaint is self-limiting
- [ ] **D** Do not make a supply. Advise the patient to drink plenty of fluids
- [ ] **E** Do not make a supply. Tell the patient to stop taking her carbimazole and seek urgent medical attention

11 Mrs Q has just been diagnosed with vaginal atrophy and her GP would like to commence her on a topical medicine. The GP seeks your advice about starting estradiol 10 mcg pessaries for Mrs Q. Which of the following does not contraindicate the use of this product?

- [ ] **A** history of breast cancer
- [ ] **B** recurrent deep vein thrombosis
- [ ] **C** unstable angina
- [ ] **D** uterine fibroids
- [ ] **E** vaginal bleeding of unknown cause

12 Mr N has been admitted to your emergency department with vomiting, fatigue and palpitations. You review the blood results in his case notes and find the following:

Parameter	Value today	Value before starting CHOP regimen
Potassium (mmol/L)	7.1	4.7
Phosphate (mmol/L)	4.7	1.2
Calcium (mmol/L)	0.7	2.3
Sodium (mmol/L)	140	135
Uric acid (mmol/L)	0.73	0.41
Serum creatinine (μmol/L)	185	96

Whilst taking his history you find that he has recently been commenced on the CHOP chemotherapy regimen for stage IV non-Hodgkin's lymphoma.

You decide to talk to the medical team urgently as you believe the patient may be suffering from which of the following conditions?

- ☐ A chemotherapy-induced gastritis
- ☐ B oral mucositis
- ☐ C tumour lysis syndrome
- ☐ D type 2 respiratory failure
- ☐ E urothelial toxicity

13 Miss Z has been diagnosed with iron deficiency anaemia, for which she received an infusion of 1000 mg *Ferinject* (ferric carboxymaltose) this morning. She now presents to your pharmacy with a prescription for ferrous sulfate tablets 200 mg TDS.
Which of the following pieces of information do you NOT need to give Miss Z?

- ☐ A Do not start taking the ferrous sulfate for another 5 days
- ☐ B Ferrous sulfate may make her constipated
- ☐ C Ferrous sulfate may turn her stools dark or black
- ☐ D She will need to take ferrous sulfate for about 2 months
- ☐ E Take the ferrous sulfate on an empty stomach

14 You are working in the hospital dispensary and receive a discharge prescription for 'methotrexate tablets, orally, 15 mg once weekly on Wednesdays'. Which of the following would be the most appropriate supply to provide 4 weeks' treatment?

- ☐ A four 10 mg tablets and eight 2.5 mg tablets
- ☐ B six 10 mg tablets
- ☐ C eighteen 2.5 mg tablets
- ☐ D twenty-four 2.5 mg tablets
- ☐ E none of the above is appropriate as the dose should be every day

15 Mr I comes into your community pharmacy with his 18-month-old son, Brady, who woke up this morning with itchy, running, eyes. He would like some advice on what this might be and what can be done about it. You look at Brady's eyes and notice that it is affecting both of his eyes, the blood vessels in the corners of his eyes are more prominent, and the sclera appears pink. The discharge seems to be watery and Mr I confirms it has not been sticky. Brady does not have a temperature and does not appear to be in any pain.
Which of the following is the most appropriate course of action to take?

☐ A   Advise Mr I to bathe and clean Brady's eyelid margins with freshly boiled and cooled water
☐ B   Supply chloramphenicol 0.5% eye drops and advise to apply every 2 hours for the first 48 hours, then every 4 hours thereafter
☐ C   Supply chloramphenicol 1% eye ointment and advise to apply every 6 hours
☐ D   Supply sodium cromoglicate 2% eye drops and advise to apply every 6 hours
☐ E   Advise Mr I to take Brady to their GP or an urgent care centre

16   Mrs L comes into your community to ask your advice regarding some chlorhexidine mouthwash you dispensed for her 2 days ago. She is complaining of stinging in her mouth during and shortly after using the product. You ask to look in her mouth and observe reddening of the gums and slight peeling of the epithelium of her cheeks.
Which of the following is the most appropriate action to take?

☐ A   Advise Mrs L to continue with the current treatment as it should be transient
☐ B   Advise Mrs L to dilute the mouthwash in an equal volume of water
☐ C   Refer Mrs L to her dentist
☐ D   Refer Mrs L to her GP
☐ E   Refer Mrs L to the urgent care centre or emergency department

17   Mr W comes into your pharmacy with a prescription for miconazole oral gel to treat oral candidiasis, which his GP believes has been caused by his poor inhaler technique. Whilst clinically appraising the prescription you look at his PMR.
Which of the following medicines would trigger you to discuss this treatment with his GP?

☐ A   aspirin
☐ B   bisoprolol
☐ C   furosemide
☐ D   ramipril
☐ E   warfarin

18 You are supplying Miss H with a tub of *Hydromol* cream (isopropyl myristate 50 mg/g, liquid paraffin 100 mg/g, sodium lactate 10 mg/g and sodium pidolate 25 mg/g) as an emollient for her dry skin, but you find that she has not used it before and has not been advised how to use it.
Which of the following is the most appropriate advice to give Miss H?

□ A Apply immediately after showering. Apply against the direction of hair growth

□ B Apply immediately after showering. Apply in the same direction of hair growth

□ C Apply immediately before showering. Apply against the direction of hair growth

□ D Apply immediately before showering. Apply in the same direction of hair growth

□ E Apply before going to bed at night. Apply in the same direction of hair growth

19 You are reviewing a patient on your trauma unit, Mr S, who was recently in a motorcycling accident and has suffered a fractured skull due to a penetrating head injury.
Which of the following vaccines should you ensure that the patient has received?

□ A Bacillus Calmette–Guérin (BCG) vaccine

□ B hepatitis B vaccine

□ C japanese encephalitis vaccine

□ D meningococcal ACWY vaccine

□ E pneumococcal (23-valent) polysaccharide vaccine

20 Mrs K has recently recovered from an episode of shingles but has been complaining of pain ever since. Her GP has diagnosed her with post-herpetic neuralgia, for which she has been prescribed *Versatis* (lidocaine 5%) medicated plasters.
Which of the following is the most appropriate action to take?

□ A Supply the product and advise her to apply once daily to a dry, non-hairy area of skin for up to 12 hours each day, ensuring a 12-hour plaster-free period

□ B Supply the product and advise her to apply each morning to a dry, non-hairy area of skin and remove before going to bed, ensuring a plaster-free period overnight

   ☐ C   Supply the product and advise her to apply once daily to a moist, non-hairy area of skin for up to 12 hours each day, ensuring a 12-hour plaster-free period

   ☐ D   Supply the product and advise her to apply each morning to a moist, non-hairy area of skin and remove before going to bed, ensuring a plaster free-period overnight

   ☐ E   Do not supply the product as it is not safe to use in post-herpetic neuralgia

21 One of the nurses on your ward comes to ask your advice regarding the administration of phenytoin to one of her patients, Mrs R, who has been prescribed a rapid loading dose of 700 mg by IV infusion. The medical team have expressed concern about her fluid balance and want to restrict Mrs R's fluid intake as much as possible. However, they are keen that she receives this dose in the shortest time possible.

What is the most appropriate administration advice to give to the nurse? You may use the SPC for phenytoin IV to help you: www.medicines.org .uk/emc/medicine/650

   ☐ A   Draw up 14 mL of the undiluted product and give as a bolus over about 3–5 minutes

   ☐ B   Draw up 14 mL of the undiluted product and infuse over 14 minutes

   ☐ C   Make the dose up to a final volume of 50 mL in 0.9% sodium chloride and infuse over 14 minutes

   ☐ D   Make the dose up to a final volume of 70 mL in 0.9% sodium chloride and infuse over 14 minutes

   ☐ E   Make the dose up to a final volume of 100 mL in 0.9% sodium chloride and infuse over 14 minutes

22 Mr V has been admitted to your emergency department with possible paracetamol overdose after taking too many cough and cold remedies, alongside paracetamol tablets around 6 hours ago. His plasma paracetamol concentration is reported as 82 mg/L.

Which of the following would be the most appropriate to prescribe for Mr V?

   ☐ A   acetylcysteine

   ☐ B   activated carbon

   ☐ C   atropine

   ☐ D   diazepam

   ☐ E   ethanol

23 You are the on-call pharmacist for your hospital and receive a call from the junior medic on call who has just been to see a patient, Mrs O, who has an infected pressure sore. The medic wants to prescribe a dressing and describes the wound as heavily exuding with a significant amount of pus.
Which of the following dressings would be the LEAST appropriate to use?

☐ A   *Algisite Ag* (alginate dressing with silver)
☐ B   *Allevyn* (foam dressing)
☐ C   *Aquacel* (hydrocolloid fibre dressing)
☐ D   *Intrasite* (hydrogel dressing)
☐ E   *Sorbsan* (alginate dressing)

24 Mr A is a 73-year-old man on your ward who has been admitted with a urinary tract infection. On the ward round the consultant wants to initiate Mr A on IV co-amoxiclav until the culture results are back. You check his laboratory results and note that his eGFR is 21 mL/min.
Which of the following dosage regimens is most appropriate to prescribe in this situation?
You may use the SPC for intravenous co-amoxiclav to help you:
http://www.medicines.org.uk/emc/medicine/32019

☐ A   500/100 mg every 12 hours
☐ B   500/100 mg every 24 hours
☐ C   1000/200 mg STAT, then 500/100 mg every 12 hours
☐ D   1000/200 mg STAT, then 500/100 mg every 24 hours
☐ E   1000/200 mg every 12 hours

25 You receive a call from a local nursing home regarding one of their residents who is now receiving end-of-life care. As a result they want to transfer the patient on to a syringe driver. You confirm that the pre-scribed drugs are compatible together in a syringe driver, but the nurse also wants to know what diluent to use to make the syringe up to an appropriate volume.
Which of the following is the most appropriate diluent to use?

☐ A   glucose 5%
☐ B   glucose 10%
☐ C   sodium chloride 0.45%
☐ D   sodium chloride 0.9%
☐ E   water for injections

26 Mr D, a 93-year-old man, has been admitted to your ward for care of older people after a fall. Whilst looking at his notes you see he has had around five falls in the last year and the medical team are concerned as these appear to be non-mechanical falls.

Which of the following of Mr D's medicines is most likely to increase his risk of falls and should therefore be reviewed or stopped?

☐ **A** alendronic acid
☐ **B** calcium carbonate with cholecalciferol
☐ **C** galantamine
☐ **D** tamsulosin
☐ **E** warfarin

27 You are working for your local prescribing support team and are asked to write PGDs (patient group directions) for the supply and administration of adrenaline pre-filled disposal pens to patients, from community pharmacies, in emergency situations.

Which of the following sections is NOT legally required to be included in the PGD?

☐ **A** Signature from patients who qualify for the PGD
☐ **B** Specific description of which patients are excluded from the PGD
☐ **C** Specific situation(s) in which the PGD can be used
☐ **D** Specification of the healthcare profession(s) that can use the PGD
☐ **E** Start date of the PGD

28 You are reviewing the latest evidence on the treatment of *C. difficile* infection and see the following forest plot from a recently published systematic review of two new antibiotics.

From the data given here, which of the following statements is true?

☐ **A** Antibiotic 2 is better at achieving bacteriological cure compared with antibiotic 1. Antibiotic 2 is better at achieving symptomatic cure compared with antibiotic 1
☐ **B** Antibiotic 2 is better at achieving bacteriological cure compared with antibiotic 1. Antibiotic 1 is better at achieving symptomatic cure compared with antibiotic 2
☐ **C** Antibiotic 2 is no better at achieving bacteriological cure compared with antibiotic 1. Antibiotic 2 is better at achieving symptomatic cure compared with antibiotic 1

☐ D   Antibiotic 2 is no better at achieving bacteriological cure compared with antibiotic 1. Antibiotic 1 is better at achieving symptomatic cure compared with antibiotic 2

☐ E   Antibiotic 1 and antibiotic 2 are equally effective at achieving symptomatic and bacteriological cure

Study	Abx1 n/N	Abx 2 n/N	Risk ratio (95% CI)	Weight	Risk ratio (95% CI)
Symptomatic Cure					
Trial 1	200/300	250/300		60%	0.85 (0.80, 0.95)
Trial 2	50/60	40/60		12%	1.15 (0.85, 1.40)
Trial 3	25/40	25/40		8%	1.00 (0.75, 1.30)
Trial 4	50/100	70/100		20%	0.80 (0.65, 0.90)
Total Z = 2.60 (P = 0.007)	**500**	**500**	◆	**100%**	**0.90 (0.85, 0.95)**
Bacteriological cure					
Trial 5	20/50	30/50		25%	0.85 (0.55, 1.20)
Trial 6	14/30	15/30		15%	0.90 (0.60, 1.60)
Trial 7	60/120	65/120		60%	0.80 (0.50, 1.10)
Total Z = 1.60 (P = 0.700)	**200**	**200**	◆	**100%**	**0.90 (0.70, 1.15)**
			Favours Abx 2 ┃ Favours Abx 1		

29 Mr Y has been taking co-beneldopa for Parkinson's disease for around 6 months, but has started to experience nausea after a recent dose increase. His GP asks you which antiemetic would be the best option to try first line.

Which of the following drugs would be the most appropriate to recommend?

☐ A   cyclizine
☐ B   domperidone
☐ C   hyoscine
☐ D   metoclopramide
☐ E   ondansetron

30 Wendy is a 3-year-old girl who has cystic fibrosis and is struggling to thrive. Her specialist team have prescribed pancreatin capsules to help with the absorption of dietary fats, proteins and carbohydrates.

Which of the following pieces of advice about pancreatin capsules is INCORRECT?

☐ **A**   Irritation of the perianal region is an indication of excessive dosing

☐ **B**   Gloves should be worn if they open the capsules

☐ **C**   The capsules and their contents should not be chewed or crushed

☐ **D**   The contents of the capsules can be mixed with hot food or fluid

☐ **E**   The contents of the capsules can be mixed with soft food or apple sauce

SECTION B

Simon Harris

1   You have read an interesting study on the use of a new medicine which has been launched for asthma, which describes the study as:

'This was an epidemiological study which describes the characteristics of a population, where data was collected at one point in time and the relationships between characteristics were considered.'

Which of the following study types does this most likely describe?

☐ **A**   case series
☐ **B**   cohort study
☐ **C**   cross-sectional study
☐ **D**   longitudinal study
☐ **E**   prospective observational study

2   Mrs R was diagnosed with schizophrenia 3 years ago, and her olanzapine 20 mg daily is no longer controlling her symptoms. She was unresponsive to risperidone and so a decision has been made for Mrs R to begin treatment with clozapine. Neutropenia, potentially fatal agranulocytosis, myocarditis and intestinal obstruction are all conditions to be aware of when initiating patients on clozapine.

Regarding agranulocytosis, which of the following tests should be carried out prior Mrs R's treatment with clozapine?

☐ **A**   creatinine clearance
☐ **B**   leucocyte and differential blood counts
☐ **C**   liver function tests
☐ **D**   random blood glucose test
☐ **E**   thyroid function test

3   You are the Responsible Pharmacist working in a busy pharmacy with two pre-registration pharmacy technicians. One of them is entering CDs in the register, and asks you whether to dispose of the recently completed CD register.

What is the minimum period of time a CD register must be kept?

☐ **A**   1 year from the date of the last entry
☐ **B**   2 years from the date of the first entry

□ C   2 years from the date of the last entry
□ D   5 years from the date of the last entry
□ E   7 years from the date of the first entry

4   Miss T, a 78-year-old woman, is taking the following medication:

- atorvastatin 40 mg daily
- clopidogrel 75 mg daily
- lansoprazole 15 mg daily
- metformin 500 mg three times daily
- ramipril 2.5 mg daily

She has type 2 diabetes and had a TIA 1 year ago. Miss T has just been diagnosed with AF and will be commencing rivaroxaban 20 mg daily. Which of Miss T's existing medication should be stopped due to commencement of rivaroxaban?

□ A   atorvastatin
□ B   clopidogrel
□ C   lansoprazole
□ D   metformin
□ E   ramipril

5   Every pharmacy professional has a duty to raise any concerns about individuals, actions or circumstances that may be unacceptable, and could result in risks to patient and public safety.
Which of the following statements does NOT reflect the GPhC's guidance on raising concerns?

□ A   Failure to raise concerns about poor practice could result in harm to patients
□ B   If you do not report any concerns you have about a colleague or others, it would be a breach of the GPhC Standards of conduct, ethics and performance
□ C   You do not have a responsibility to raise concerns if you are a locum or temporary staff
□ D   You should keep a record of the concerns you have, who you have raised them with and the response or action that has been taken as a result of your actions
□ E   If your concern is about a specific person, e.g. a patient or colleague, you should, where possible, maintain confidentiality

6   Mrs O is taking ethinylestradiol as a means to alleviate her menopausal symptoms; however, she is worried about the risks and side-effects that come with hormonal replacement therapy.
Which of the following adverse effects is NOT a reason to stop her medication immediately?

  □ A   a blood pressure reading of 145/90 mmHg
  □ B   severe stomach pain
  □ C   sudden, severe chest pain
  □ D   swelling in the calf of one leg
  □ E   unusual, severe, prolonged headache

7   Mr H has been prescribed domperidone to relieve his nausea, and hands you his prescription to be dispensed. When giving out his medication, Mr H explains that he has never taken it before and would like to know more about his medication before he begins taking it.
Which of the following statements regarding advice on domperidone is CORRECT?

  □ A   Domperidone should be used at the highest effective dose for the shortest possible duration
  □ B   Maximum treatment duration with domperidone should not normally exceed 7 days
  □ C   Domperidone is associated with a small increased risk of developing certain types of cancer
  □ D   The recommended dose in adults is 5 mg up to four times daily
  □ E   The maximum daily dose of domperidone is 20 mg

8   New alcohol guidelines were produced in January 2016, partly because of the increased evidence of the link between alcohol and cancer, and partly because the previous guidelines were released in 1995, and the science has changed significantly since then.
Which of the following statements regarding alcohol consumption is INCORRECT?

  □ A   Drinking alcohol even at low levels contributes to a wide range of health harms, to a range of diseases and to hospital admissions
  □ B   If a person drinks 14 units of alcohol per week, they are best to spread it evenly over 2 days or more
  □ C   It is safest not to regularly drink more than 14 units of alcohol per week

☐ D   It is safest to avoid drinking alcohol altogether in pregnancy

☐ E   There is an increased risk at low levels of alcohol consumption for breast, oesophageal, oral cavity cancer and cancer of the pharynx

9   A patient comes into your pharmacy and hands you a prescription for his anti-epileptic medication. You notice that the prescriber has issued the medication by the brand name, and you inform the patient that you will need to order more stock as you do not currently hold the specific brand stated on the prescription.
Which of the following anti-epileptic medicines listed below must be dispensed using a specific brand agreed by the prescriber?

☐ A   clonazepam

☐ B   gabapentin

☐ C   levetiracetam

☐ D   phenytoin

☐ E   pregabalin

10   When delivering health promotion activities and giving advice to patients in the pharmacy, it can be useful to consider the five stages of behaviour change. By doing so, pharmacy staff are able to hold more appropriate conversations with patients, which are ultimately more likely to lead to a positive change in behaviour.
Which of the following is NOT one of the five stages of behaviour change?

☐ A   action

☐ B   contemplation

☐ C   maintenance

☐ D   preparation

☐ E   reflection

11   Rapid detection and recording of adverse drug reactions (ADRs) is of vital importance so that unrecognised hazards are identified promptly and appropriate regulatory action is taken to ensure that medicines are used safely. Suspected ADRs should be reported directly to the MHRA through the Yellow Card Scheme.
Which of the following statements regarding the reporting of ADRs via the Yellow Card Scheme is INCORRECT?

☐ A   All effects on fertility should be reported

☐ B   All endocrine disturbances should be reported

☐ C   Any drug interactions which cause an adverse effect should be reported

☐ D   Any reaction in the elderly should be reported

☐ E   Any reaction which prolongs hospitalisation should be reported

12 Mr K has been admitted to hospital following a fall at home. He has been prescribed a parenteral anticoagulant for the prevention of venous thromboembolism, and the doctor has selected tinzaparin, based on local guidelines.

Which of the following reasons for prescribing a low-molecular-weight heparin (LMWH) rather than unfractionated heparin is CORRECT?

☐ A   LMWH are preferred for use in patients at high risk of bleeding

☐ B   LMWH have greater anticoagulant monitoring requirements, and therefore clinicians have more control over their effects

☐ C   LMWH have a short duration of action and therefore its effect can be terminated rapidly if needed

☐ D   LMWH allow patients to have regular INR monitoring to ensure a safe blood concentration

☐ E   LMWH have a lower risk of heparin-induced thrombocytopenia

13 Mr S is a 68-year-old patient with a past medical history of atrial fibrillation and stroke. He has been on warfarin for about 3 years and has been on a stable dose. Last week, however, he suffered a seizure and was admitted to hospital, where he was prescribed an anti-epileptic drug. Today his INR is 1.7 (target 2–3).

Which of the following medicines is most likely to be responsible for the decrease in his INR?

☐ A   carbamazepine

☐ B   diazepam

☐ C   gabapentin

☐ D   pregabalin

☐ E   valproate

14 The General Pharmaceutical Council (GPhC) recently launched new standards for pharmacy professionals, which came into effect on 12 May 2017. All pharmacy professionals in Great Britain are required to meet these standards, which describe how safe and effective care

is delivered, and help pharmacy professionals to demonstrate their professionalism and deliver person-centred care. Pharmacy owners also have a responsibility to make sure that they are creating and supporting an environment in which pharmacy professionals can meet these standards.

Which of the following statements on the new GPhC standards is INCORRECT?

- ☐ A The standards are relevant to all pharmacy students and trainees while they are on their journey towards registration and practice
- ☐ B Pharmacy professionals are personally accountable for meeting the standards and must be able to justify the decisions they make
- ☐ C The standards apply and must be met at all times only during working hours
- ☐ D There are nine standards that every pharmacy professional is accountable for meeting
- ☐ E The standards apply to all pharmacists and pharmacy technicians

15 You are running a workshop in a local community centre on diet and exercise. One participant tells you that she is slightly overweight with a BMI of 26, and she believes a lack of exercise is mostly responsible for this weight gain. Another participant then tells you that he has a 4-year-old daughter and is worried that she too is not doing enough physical activity. She has no physical or mental disabilities, and the father is wondering how much exercise his daughter should be doing.

Which of the following statements is the MOST appropriate advice to give him regarding exercise for his 4-year-old daughter?

- ☐ A Levels of physical activity do not need to be monitored until children reach their teenage years
- ☐ B Children aged <12 should be physically active for at least 1 hour a day
- ☐ C Children aged <5 should be physically active every day for at least 3 hours a day
- ☐ D If a parent is concerned their child is not active enough, they should restrict their intake of fatty foods to prevent weight gain
- ☐ E Children aged <18 should aim to achieve at least 150 minutes of moderate intensity activity per week

16 The veterinary cascade is a process which allows the prescribing and supply of medicines which are not licensed for animals.

Which of the following CANNOT be supplied under the terms of the veterinary cascade?

☐ **A** A veterinary medicinal product authorised in the UK for another species or different condition

☐ **B** A product prepared extemporaneously by a registered pharmacist in accordance with a veterinary prescription

☐ **C** A licensed human medicine

☐ **D** An unlicensed veterinary medicine in the EU

☐ **E** A licensed human medicine not authorised in the UK but authorised in another European Union country

17 Whilst working in a pharmacy, you are made aware of a dispensing error in which amlodipine 10 mg was given to a patient instead of bisoprolol 10 mg. You check the pharmacy record and notice that you were the Responsible Pharmacist on the day the error was made. The patient has come to the pharmacy to make an official complaint and to find out who was responsible.

In the case of dispensing errors and complaints, which of the following statements is INCORRECT?

☐ **A** You should empathise with the patient's situation, but not offer an apology before a full investigation and root cause analysis has been completed

☐ **B** You should inform your professional indemnity insurance provider of the error

☐ **C** You should provide details of how to make an official complaint if requested

☐ **D** You should ask to inspect the incorrect medicine

☐ **E** You should establish if the patient has taken any of the incorrect medicine

18 The introduction of a statutory Duty of Candour was a major step towards implementing a key recommendation from the Francis Inquiry. Which of the following statements most accurately describes the professional duty of candour?

☐ **A** As a pharmacist, you should request that a colleague does not raise a concern about another pharmacist if you believe this may put their registration at risk

☐ **B** The professional duty of candour is listed as one of the seven principles of conduct, ethics and performance, and involves developing your professional knowledge and competence

□ C   Every healthcare professional must be open and honest with patients when something goes wrong with their treatment or care, including offering an apology and appropriate remedy or support if possible, to put matters right

□ D   Candour refers to recognising diversity and respecting people's cultural differences and their right to hold their personal values and beliefs

□ E   Candour refers to recognising the limits of your professional competence, and practising only in those areas in which you are competent to do so

19 Before disclosing confidential information, you must ensure you have considered all relevant factors.
    Which of the following is NOT required when disclosing confidential information?

□ A   Disclosing only the information needed for the particular purpose

□ B   Justifying your decisions and any actions you take

□ C   Making appropriate records to show who the request came from, whether the patient's consent was obtained, whether consent was given or refused, and what information was disclosed

□ D   Obtaining the patient's consent even if disclosure is required by law

□ E   Releasing information promptly once you are satisfied what information should be disclosed, having taken all necessary steps to protect confidentiality

20 A 16-year-old boy has been prescribed isotretinoin 20 mg capsules once daily for 1 month. You see on his medical record that he was also prescribed omeprazole capsules OD 2 months ago, and he tells you he currently takes *Gaviscon* liquid PRN and multivitamins A–Z OD.
    Which of the following is the most appropriate counselling advice to give this patient?

□ A   He should stop taking the *Gaviscon* liquid as it will interact with the isotretinoin

□ B   He should take the isotretinoin as prescribed as there are no interactions with any of the other medicines that he is currently taking

□ C   He should stop taking the multivitamins as they contain vitamin A

☐ **D**   He should not take the omeprazole and *Gaviscon* together
☐ **E**   He should avoid indigestion remedies whilst taking the isotretinoin capsules

21   Miss L has brought her 4-week-old baby boy to the pharmacy. She has a prescription to treat her recurring skin condition, and explains she would like you to check whether the antibiotic is safe to take whilst breast-feeding.
Which of the following antibiotics would be the LEAST appropriate for Miss L?

☐ **A**   cephalexin
☐ **B**   co-amoxiclav
☐ **C**   erythromycin
☐ **D**   lymecycline
☐ **E**   penicillin V

22   Mrs W, a 19-year-old patient of yours, explains to you that she has been suffering from menorrhagia for the last 2 months. She recently received advice from a friend regarding tranexamic acid tablets and their availability over the counter.
Which of the following statements about the use of over-the-counter tranexamic acid is CORRECT?

☐ **A**   Tranexamic acid belongs to a group of medicines called fibrinolytics
☐ **B**   Tranexamic acid would not be appropriate for Mrs W as it is only licensed for women aged 21–45 years
☐ **C**   Tranexamic acid should be taken for a maximum of 4 consecutive days
☐ **D**   The dose for menorrhagia is two 500 mg tablets three times a day for the duration of the period
☐ **E**   Mrs W should be advised that common side-effects include nausea, vomiting and diarrhoea, which can be resolved by increasing the dose

23   Miss P regularly asks you to order St John's wort tablets for her. She's been using the same brand for the last 4 years and finds them very effective. Four months ago she went through a difficult divorce and, after discussing the stress and anxiety of this with her GP, she has been prescribed citalopram 10 mg OD. Her GP advised her to take these for 1 month and then return for a review. Miss P tells you that she forgot to ask her GP if it was OK to continue taking the St John's wort tablets alongside the citalopram. What of the following is the most appropriate advice to give Miss P regarding her citalopram tablets?

- ☐ A   She should take the citalopram tablets with a full glass of water to ensure they dissolve completely in the stomach
- ☐ B   St John's wort is more effective than citalopram 10 mg, so she may therefore prefer to increase her dose rather than begin a new medication
- ☐ C   St John's wort interacts with citalopram so it's best to stop taking it before she begins the citalopram
- ☐ D   St John's wort has a positive interaction with citalopram, in that the two tablets together will provide a synergistic effect, and they can be safely taken together
- ☐ E   It is best to take St John's wort and citalopram tablets on alternate days for the first month until her next review with her GP

24 Mrs K has come to your pharmacy with her 30-month-old son. She explains that he's been feeling quite uncomfortable around his bottom area for the last few days, and has been scratching at it a lot, especially at night. You explain to Mrs K that the symptoms she is describing sound like threadworms.
Which of the following is the most appropriate advice to give Mrs K?

- ☐ A   Explain that threadworms are common in young children, and that no treatment is required as threadworms survive in the body only for 2 weeks
- ☐ B   Refer Mrs K to her GP as there are no over-the-counter treatments available for her son due to his age
- ☐ C   Offer calamine lotion for the itching, and advise her to regularly wash her son's linen to prevent re-infection
- ☐ D   Offer mebendazole chewable tablets for her son, and explain that all members of her family will require treatment to prevent re-infection
- ☐ E   Offer permethrin cream, and advise her to apply the cream to her son's bottom once daily for 7 days

25 Mr G has come to your pharmacy to buy paracetamol 120 mg/5 mL suspension for his 8-month-old baby boy. He has recently starting teething, and Mr G thinks he has a mild temperature.

Which of the following is the most appropriate dose for Mr G's son?

- ☐ **A** 2.5 mL every 6–8 hours (max. 4 doses in 24 hours)
- ☐ **B** 60 mg every 4–6 hours (max. 6 doses in 24 hours)
- ☐ **C** 5 mL every 4–6 hours (max. 4 doses in 24 hours)
- ☐ **D** 120 mg every 6–8 hours (max. 6 doses in 24 hours)
- ☐ **E** 7.5 mL every 4–6 hours (max. 4 doses in 24 hours)

26 Mr C enters your pharmacy to purchase some multivitamin supplements. He takes orlistat 120 mg TDS and is aware that orlistat can affect the absorption of fat-soluble vitamins. He would like to know which vitamins are fat soluble.
Which of the following vitamins is NOT fat soluble?

- ☐ **A** vitamin A
- ☐ **B** vitamin B
- ☐ **C** vitamin D
- ☐ **D** vitamin E
- ☐ **E** vitamin K

27 You are running a workshop to advise patients how to use different medical devices.
Which of the following statements is CORRECT?

- ☐ **A** Eye ointment should be applied as a thin line inside the lower eyelid
- ☐ **B** Patients should tilt their head forward when administering nose drops
- ☐ **C** In order to minimise side-effects, patients should be advised to blow their nose after using a nasal spray
- ☐ **D** Buccal tablets should be placed under the tongue and allowed to dissolve
- ☐ **E** When using dry powder inhalers, breathe in slowly and deeply through the mouthpiece

28 Mrs A is collecting her new prescription for sublingual glyceryl trinitrate (GTN) 300-mcg tablets, which has been prescribed for her angina. Mrs A has never used them before and therefore requires further information on how best to take them.
Which of the following counselling points for Mrs A about her new tablets is INCORRECT?

- ☐ **A** Sublingual GTN tablets provide rapid symptomatic relief of angina, but its effects last only 5–10 minutes

☐ **B** GTN tablets should be discarded 8 weeks after opening
☐ **C** GTN tablets should preferably be taken sitting down
☐ **D** GTN tablets should not be transferred to another container
☐ **E** Facial flushing may occur as a side effect after taking GTN tablets

29 Miss E asks you to recommend a suitable treatment for a rash on her arm. After examining her arm and questioning Miss E you suspect she has ringworm. Miss E seems surprised when you tell her and asks what exactly ringworm is.
Which of the following should you advise Miss E that ringworm is?

☐ **A** a bacterial infection
☐ **B** a fungal infection
☐ **C** a viral infection
☐ **D** an infestation with parasitic worms
☐ **E** an infestation with mites

30 Mrs V takes isoniazid as part of her treatment regimen for tuberculosis. When she presents her prescription she asks you why she has also been prescribed pyridoxine.
Which of the following adverse effects of isoniazid can be prevented by the prophylactic use of pyridoxine?

☐ **A** agranulocytosis
☐ **B** hepatitis
☐ **C** nausea
☐ **D** peripheral neuropathy
☐ **E** skin rash

31 A patient receives amikacin 500 mg by IM injection TDS for a soft-tissue infection (target range for amikacin: peak <30 mg/L, trough <10 mg/L). Three days later a peak amikacin level of 29 mg/L is reported, with a trough concentration of 14 mg/L.
Which of the following is an appropriate method of dose rationalisation?

☐ **A** Decrease the dose and decrease the dosage interval
☐ **B** Increase the dose and increase the dosage interval
☐ **C** Increase the dose and maintain the same dosage interval
☐ **D** Maintain the same dose and increase the dosage interval
☐ **E** Maintain the same dose and decrease the dosage interval

32 Mrs J is a 51-year-old patient who was commenced on pioglitazone 15 mg OD 6 weeks ago. This was in addition to her metformin 500 mg TDS which she has been taking for the past 3 years. When collecting her repeat prescription, she complains of abdominal pain, being tired and dark urine. She wonders if the new tablet might be the cause of her symptoms.
Which of the following is the most appropriate advice for Mrs J?

- ☐ A   She should see the GP as the dose of pioglitazone may need to be reduced
- ☐ B   She should see the GP as the dose of pioglitazone may need to be increased
- ☐ C   The symptoms described are not known to be caused by pioglitazone
- ☐ D   She should stop taking pioglitazone straight away and see her GP as soon as possible
- ☐ E   She is experiencing a side-effect of pioglitazone and, although it is safe to continue taking it she may wish to see her GP for an alternative

33 Whilst ordering *Oramorph* 20 mg/1 mL concentrated solution from a wholesaler, your dispensary assistant asks you to explain the differences between the various controlled drug (CD) schedules.
Which of the following statements regarding *Oramorph* 20 mg/1 mL concentrated solution is INCORRECT?

- ☐ A   It is designated a CD POM
- ☐ B   An entry into the appropriate CD register is required on the same day as stock is received, or at the latest the following day
- ☐ C   Once expired, it must be denatured before being disposed of
- ☐ D   It must be stored in the CD cabinet
- ☐ E   Invoices must be retained for 2 years

34 Miss Y, a 61-year-old female patient, has been admitted to the acute admissions unit. You are checking her medical records and note that her eGFR is 25 mL/min per 1.73m^2.
What degree of renal impairment does Miss Y have?

- ☐ A   normal
- ☐ B   mild
- ☐ C   moderate

☐ **D** severe
☐ **E** established renal failure

35 Whilst working in a GP practice, the GP Registrar calls you for some advice. She has a young patient with Parkinson's disease who requires treatment for nausea. The patient has no other medical conditions.
Which of the following antiemetics would be the most appropriate to recommend?

☐ **A** cinnarizine
☐ **B** domperidone
☐ **C** granisetron
☐ **D** metoclopramide
☐ **E** prochlorperazine

36 A patient brings in a prescription for lithium 200 mg MR tablets. You notice from your PMR that they have never been to your pharmacy before and, after talking to the patient, you discover that this is the first time they've been prescribed this medication.
Which of the following counselling points regarding lithium 200 mg MR tablets is INCORRECT?

☐ **A** The patient should maintain an adequate fluid intake
☐ **B** The patient should avoid dietary changes that may increase or decrease K^+ levels
☐ **C** The patient should report polyuria or polydipsia
☐ **D** The patient should report persistent headaches or visual disturbance
☐ **E** The patient should use effective contraception during treatment to avoid pregnancy

37 When providing a seasonal influenza vaccination service, pharmacists must be trained to respond appropriately in the event that a patient has an anaphylactic reaction.
Which of the following is the appropriate dose of adrenaline for a 6-year-old child?

☐ **A** 0.15 mL of a 1 mg/1 mL injection
☐ **B** 150 mcg
☐ **C** 0.3 mL of a 1 in 1000 injection
☐ **D** 0.5 mL of a 1 mg/1 mL injection
☐ **E** 750 mcg

38 There is a statutory requirement for pharmacists to record their continuing professional development (CPD). The GPhC specifies the amount of CPD to be completed during each year of registration. They also state that CPD entries must be relevant to the safe and effective practice of pharmacy and your own scope of practice.
Which of the following statements regarding CPD is CORRECT?

☐ A You must record a maximum of nine CPD entries per registration year

☐ B The criteria for the review of CPD records require you to submit nine entries completed for each full review period, with five of these starting at the reflection phase of the CPD cycle

☐ C The GPhC CPD cycle consists of the following four phased learning process: Reflection, Planning, Action and Evaluation

☐ D For pharmacists working part time, you can apply to the GPhC to reduce the amount of CPD that is required each year

☐ E You are not expected to cover the full scope of your practice in your CPD record, and have the option of selecting the roles that you spend most your time in to write about

39 Pharmacists should be familiar with the risk of developmental disorders in children born to mothers who take sodium valproate during pregnancy. To ensure female patients are aware of these risks, the MHRA have produced a toolkit that includes information for patients and prescribers.
Which of the following pieces of advice would NOT be appropriate to give when dispensing valproate for female patients?

☐ A Advise patients how to recognise the signs and symptoms of blood or liver disorders and pancreatitis, and to seek medical attention if these develop

☐ B If there is an unplanned pregnancy whilst a patient is taking valproate medicines, advise the patient to stop treatment and arrange to see their prescriber urgently to review treatment

☐ C Patients should be advised that it is not recommended to drink alcohol whilst taking valproate medicines

☐ D Remind patients to avoid abrupt withdrawal

☐ E Women of child-bearing age who are using valproate medicines should be advised on the use of effective contraception

40 Miss N, a 23-year-old female patient, has come into your pharmacy with a prescription for isotretinoin. Miss N is under the pregnancy prevention programme (PPP) and, after completing your checks, you decide to supply the medication to her.

Which of the following statements is CORRECT regarding the supply of oral isotretinoin and the pregnancy prevention programme (PPP)?

☐ A   All female patients need to be on the PPP when starting oral isotretinoin

☐ B   The PPP should be in place during treatment to protect female patients from pregnancy, and should continue for at least 6 weeks after stopping oral isotretinoin

☐ C   Under the PPP, prescriptions are valid for only 14 days. Prescriptions presented after 14 days should be considered expired

☐ D   For all patients on isotretinoin, a maximum of 30 days' supply can be given

☐ E   Conjunctivitis is a very common side-effect of taking oral isotretinoin

SECTION C

Questions 1–5 concern Mrs B, a White British patient, who has been prescribed lisinopril 5 mg tablets. The summary of product characteristics can be accessed here: https://www.medicines.org.uk/emc/medicine/23997

1 Mrs B is worried about taking these tablets. Her brother also takes them and developed pancreatitis. Mrs B would like to know the possibility that these tablets could cause her to develop pancreatitis.
   Which one of the following is correct regarding the possibility that these tablets could cause pancreatitis?

   - ☐ **A** $\geq 10\%$
   - ☐ **B** $\geq 1\%, <10\%$
   - ☐ **C** $\geq 0.1\%, <1\%$
   - ☐ **D** $\geq 0.1\%, <0.01\%$
   - ☐ **E** $<0.01\%$

2 Mrs B also takes a number of other medicines as well as the newly initiated lisinopril 5 mg tablets.
   Which one of the medicines taken by Mrs B, listed below, may undergo an enhanced effect with concomitant use of lisinopril 5 mg tablets?

   - ☐ **A** amitriptyline
   - ☐ **B** cimetidine
   - ☐ **C** co-codamol
   - ☐ **D** conjugated oestrogens 0.625 mg
   - ☐ **E** lithium

3 What is the most appropriate piece of counselling advice the pharmacist should give the patient from the list below?

   - ☐ **A** This medicine may cause you to feel tired; it is very common
   - ☐ **B** This medicine may cause you to develop a rash; it is very common
   - ☐ **C** This medicine may cause you to develop a cough; it is common
   - ☐ **D** This medicine may cause diarrhoea; it is very common
   - ☐ **E** This medicine may cause you to gain weight; it is very common

4   Eighteen months have passed and Mrs B is due to have a baby in 3 weeks'
time. The doctor stopped the lisinopril whilst she was pregnant but Mrs
B is keen to take it after the baby is born as the 'new blood pressure
treatment made her feel funny'. She tells you she will also be restarting
her lithium tablets once the baby is born and wondered if it safe to
breast-feed whilst taking both tablets.
What is the most appropriate piece of advice the pharmacist should
give the patient from the list below?

    ☐ A   Both drugs are safe to take whilst breast-feeding
    ☐ B   Only lithium is safe to take whilst while breast-feeding
    ☐ C   Only lisinopril is safe to take whilst breast-feeding
    ☐ D   Neither drug is safe to take if you would like to breast-feed
    ☐ E   Take the lisinopril 3 hours before breast-feeding, so that no
          harmful effects come to the baby

5   Mrs B has a female friend whose ethnicity is Black African. She has also
developed high blood pressure and her doctor told her that lisinopril
was not suitable for her because of her ethnicity. Mrs B would like to
know why this is.
What is the most appropriate response the pharmacist should give
Mrs B from the list below?

    ☐ A   Lisinopril is less effective in the black population due to low
          levels of phosphate in black populations
    ☐ B   Lisinopril is less effective in the black population due to low
          levels of calcium in black populations
    ☐ C   Lisinopril is less effective in the black population
    ☐ D   Lisinopril is less effective in the black population due to low
          levels of potassium in black populations
    ☐ E   Lisinopril is less effective in the black population due to low
          levels of sodium in black populations

Questions 6–10 concern Mrs K who has been prescribed carvedilol
3.125 mg tablets. The summary of product characteristics for can be accessed
here: https://www.medicines.org.uk/emc/medicine/27716

6   Mrs K is worried about taking these tablets. One of her friends also
takes them and developed depression. Mrs K would like to know the
possibility that these tablets could cause her to develop depression.
Which one of the following is correct regarding the association with
the development of depression in patients taking this medicine?

☐ A ≥1/10
☐ B ≥1/100 and <1/10
☐ C ≥1/1000 and <1/100
☐ D <1/10 000
☐ E ≥1/10 000 and <1/1000

7 Mrs K also takes a number of other medicines as well as the newly initiated carvedilol 3.125 mg tablets.
Which one of the medicines taken by Mrs K, listed below, may undergo an enhanced effect with concomitant use of carvedilol 3.125 mg tablets?

☐ A beclometasone
☐ B cimetidine
☐ C conjugated oestrogens 0.625 mg
☐ D doxazosin
☐ E ibuprofen

8 What is the most appropriate piece of counselling advice the pharmacist should give the patient from the list below?

☐ A This medicine may cause you to develop anaemia; it is common
☐ B This medicine may cause you to develop thrombocytopenia; it is very rare
☐ C This medicine may cause you to develop nasal congestion; it is very common
☐ D This medicine may cause dizziness; it is common
☐ E This medicine may cause you to gain weight; it is very common

9 You have been asked to prepare a lunchtime learning session for the new GP trainees at the local surgery on heart failure, and wish to include a section on the signs and symptoms associated with medication overdosage.
What is the most appropriate piece of information to include in your presentation with regard to overdosage with carvedilol from the list below?

☐ A Symptoms and signs may include diarrhoea
☐ B Symptoms and signs may include cardiac arrest
☐ C Symptoms and signs may include severe hypertension
☐ D Symptoms and signs may include tachycardia
☐ E Symptoms and signs may include absence seizures

10 At the lunchtime training session, one of the trainees tells you that they are thinking about initiating carvedilol in one of their patients who has moderate renal impairment. They would like to know if the dose needs to be altered.

What is the most appropriate piece of advice to provide the GP trainee from the list below?

- ☐ A There is no data available on the effect this drug has in patients with renal impairment
- ☐ B The medication is contraindicated in renal impairment
- ☐ C The dose should be quartered
- ☐ D The dose should be halved
- ☐ E There is normally no need to adjust the dose of this drug in patients with renal impairment

11 Mrs G, a 57-year-old patient, comes to the community pharmacy to collect her repeat prescription. She was commenced on canagliflozin 100 mg OD 5 days ago, following a review with her GP. She tells you that she has been extremely dizzy and feels very faint when she stands up. She asks you if this could have been brought on by the new tablet. What is the most appropriate advice to give to this patient?

- ☐ A The symptoms are not known to be caused by canagliflozin
- ☐ B She should see her GP as the dose of canagliflozin may need to be increased
- ☐ C She should stop taking the canagliflozin until she sees her GP
- ☐ D She is experiencing a side-effect of canagliflozin, which is likely to disappear after continued use
- ☐ E She should see her GP as soon as possible

12 Mrs D, a 58-year-old patient, comes to the community pharmacy to collect her repeat prescription. She was commenced on alendronic acid 10 mg OD 4 days ago, following a review with her GP. She tells you that she feels pain on swallowing and has developed heartburn. She asks you if this could have been brought on by the new tablet.

What is the most appropriate advice to give to this patient?

- ☐ A The symptoms are not known to be caused by alendronic acid
- ☐ B She should see her GP the dose of alendronic acid may need to be increased

□ C   She should stop taking the alendronic acid until she sees
her GP

□ D   She is experiencing a side effect of alendronic acid, which is
likely to disappear after continued use

□ E   She should keep taking alendronic acid, but also see her GP
as soon as possible

13   Mrs F, a 58-year-old woman, is a patient on your cardiology ward. She
has coronary artery disease and was fitted with a stent a few days ago.
An hour ago she was administered a hyoscine hydrobromide injection.
You are on your ward round and she tells you that she feels as though
'her heart is racing'. She informs you this started 15 minutes ago, and
asks if this could be related to the injection she was given.
What is the most appropriate course of action to take from the list
below?

□ A   Reassure her that it is very unlikely to be an effect of the
injection

□ B   Explain that she is likely to require another hyoscine
hydrobromide injection to alleviate the symptoms she is
experiencing

□ C   Reassure her that you will tell the doctor on the ward once
you have finished your ward round

□ D   Reassure her that you will tell the nurse as you are seeing
her in her meeting in 3 hours' time

□ E   Inform the doctor on the ward straight away

Questions 14–17 concern Mr V, a 49-year-old man, who has recently been
prescribed omeprazole 20 mg capsules.
    The summary of product characteristics for omeprazole 20 mg cap-
sules can be accessed here: https://www.medicines.org.uk/emc/medicine/
32529

14   Mr V is worried about taking this medication. He has heard that taking
this medicine could cause toxic epidermal necrolysis.
    Which one of the following is correct regarding the possibility that this
medication could cause toxic epidermal necrolysis?

□ A   common
□ B   rare
□ C   uncommon
□ D   unknown
□ E   very rare

15 Mr V would like to know what symptoms he should be vigilant for if he accidentally takes too much of this medication.
Which one of the following symptoms should he be vigilant for?

   ☐ **A**   abdominal pain
   ☐ **B**   mouth irritation
   ☐ **C**   rash
   ☐ **D**   reduced libido
   ☐ **E**   tremor

16 Mr V would like to know how to store this medication.
Which one of the following best describes how this product should be stored?

   ☐ **A**   Keep in a dark place
   ☐ **B**   Keep in direct sunlight
   ☐ **C**   Protect from frost
   ☐ **D**   Protect from moisture
   ☐ **E**   Store below 35°C

17 Six months have passed and Mr V comes to the pharmacy with a prescription for amoxicillin tablets as he has developed community-acquired pneumonia.
Which one of the following is most likely to occur?

   ☐ **A**   Omeprazole levels may increase
   ☐ **B**   Omeprazole levels may decrease
   ☐ **C**   Omeprazole levels will remain unchanged
   ☐ **D**   Amoxicillin levels may increase
   ☐ **E**   Amoxicillin levels may decrease

Questions 18–22 concern Miss S, a 6-year-old girl, of normal weight for her age, who has recently been prescribed amoxicillin 250 mg/5 mL oral suspension to treat acute streptococcal tonsillitis.
   The summary of product characteristics for amoxicillin 250 mg/5 mL oral suspension can be accessed here: https://www.medicines.org.uk/emc/medicine/31832

18 Miss S's father is worried about his daughter taking this medication. He has heard that taking this medicine could cause convulsions.
Which one of the following is correct regarding the possibility that this medication could cause convulsions?

☐ A common
☐ B rare
☐ C uncommon
☐ D unknown
☐ E very rare

19 Miss S's father would like to know if he should give the medication to his daughter before she eats her meals.
Which one of the following statements best describes the response you should provide?

☐ A Amoxicillin should be administered before meals
☐ B Amoxicillin should be administered after meals
☐ C Amoxicillin should not be given with milk-containing foods
☐ D Amoxicillin should not be given with vitamin A-containing foods
☐ E You can give the medication when you feel appropriate as food does not affect it

20 Miss S's father would like to know how to store this medication now that the pharmacist has made it up with water.
Which one of the following best describes how this product should be stored?

☐ A Store at 2–8°C in the refrigerator
☐ B Store in a dark place
☐ C Store out of sunlight
☐ D Protect from moisture
☐ E Store at room temperature

21 On asking Miss S's father if his daughter is allergic to anything, he tells you that she is allergic to E131 (patent blue V).
Which one of the following best describes your course of action based on this response?

☐ A Ring the GP and recommend an alternative antibiotic
☐ B Explain to Miss S's father that he should be vigilant to see whether Miss S develops a rash
☐ C Ask Miss S's father if he has antihistamines to give to Miss S should she ever develop a reaction
☐ D Ring the GP and ask them to prescribe Miss S an adrenaline pen
☐ E There is no need to do anything

22 Miss S's father comes to the pharmacy 3 days after his daughter has commenced the antibiotic course. He tells you that he is taking Miss S to the surgery tomorrow to have her oral typhoid vaccination as they are all going on holiday to South America. He would like to know if this appointment is appropriate to continue with now that his daughter is taking amoxicillin.
   Which one of the following best describes what course of action the pharmacist should take?

   □ A   Advise that the appointment should take place as planned
   □ B   Advise that the appointment should be cancelled
   □ C   Advise that the appointment be rescheduled for when the course of treatment is complete
   □ D   Advise that the appointment is not necessary
   □ E   Advise that the appointment be rescheduled for 8 weeks' time

23 Mrs C has just brought 2-weeks' worth of unused blister packs to the pharmacy which belonged to her father who died 5 days ago. All of the tablets in the blister packs were prescription-only medicines (none were controlled drugs).
   What is the most appropriate course of action for the pharmacy to take?

   □ A   Reuse the medicine for another patient
   □ B   De-blister all the tablets and place them into a secure waste container
   □ C   Place the blister packs into a secure waste container without de-blistering
   □ D   De-blister all the tablets and place them into a yellow sharps container
   □ E   Advise Mrs C to dispose of the waste medication in her domestic waste

24 Mrs D, a 34-year-old patient, comes to the community pharmacy and asks to speak with the pharmacist. She was commenced on a combined oral contraceptive pill 4 days ago, following a review with her GP. She tells you that in the last 24 hours she has noticed that her left calf has become swollen and is causing her severe pain. She asks you if this could have been brought on by the new tablet.
   What is the most appropriate advice to give to this patient?

   □ A   The symptoms are not known to be caused by the combined oral contraceptive pill

☐ B   She should see her GP as the dose of the combined oral contraceptive pill may need to be reduced

☐ C   She should stop taking the combined oral contraceptive pill and seek medical immediately

☐ D   She is experiencing a side-effect of the combined oral contraceptive pill, which is likely to disappear after continued use

☐ E   She should keep taking the combined oral contraceptive pill, but also see her GP as soon as possible

25 Mrs F, a 52-year-old patient, comes to the community pharmacy and asks to speak with the pharmacist. She was commenced on atorvastatin 6 days ago, following a review with her GP. She tells you that, in the last 48 hours, she has noticed that her right leg feels weaker than before and that it is hurting. She asks you if this could have been brought on by the new tablet.

What is the most appropriate advice to give to this patient?

☐ A   The symptoms are not known to be caused by atorvastatin

☐ B   She should see her GP as the dose of atorvastatin may need to be reduced

☐ C   She should stop taking atorvastatin and seek medical attention as soon as possible

☐ D   She is experiencing a side-effect of atorvastatin, which is likely to disappear after continued use

☐ E   She should keep taking atorvastatin, but also see her GP as soon as possible

26 Mrs J, a 48-year-old patient has been admitted to hospital with a chest infection. She currently takes aminophylline tablets and the doctor wishes to commence her on an antibiotic. She has no known drug allergies.

Which of the following antibiotics is the most appropriate to recommend?

☐ A   amoxicillin

☐ B   ciprofloxacin

☐ C   clarithromycin

☐ D   erythromycin

☐ E   norfloxacin

27 Mrs F, a 54-year-old patient, has been commenced on ramipril tablets. She currently takes no other medication and has no known drug allergies. She would like to know if she can drink alcohol whilst taking these tablets.

Which of the following is the most appropriate response?

□ A   You are likely to feel faint if you drink alcohol and take the drug

□ B   This drug has no effect on alcohol

□ C   This drug will make your heart beat faster if you drink alcohol as well

□ D   This drug will make you feel sleepier if you drink alcohol as well

□ E   This drug will make it more difficult to breathe if you drink alcohol as well

28 Mr P, a 65-year-old patient, has been commenced on doxazosin tablets. He currently takes no other medication and has no known drug allergies. He would like to know if he can drink alcohol whilst taking these tablets.
Which of the following is the most appropriate response?

□ A   You are likely to feel faint if you drink alcohol and take the drug

□ B   This drug has no effect on alcohol

□ C   This drug will make your heart beat faster if you drink alcohol as well

□ D   This drug will make you feel sleepier if you drink alcohol as well

□ E   This drug will make it more difficult to breathe if you drink alcohol as well

29 Mrs Z, a 42-year-old patient, has been commenced on amitriptyline tablets. She currently takes no other medication and has no known drug allergies. She would like to know if she can drink alcohol whilst taking these tablets.
Which of the following is the most appropriate response?

□ A   You are likely to feel faint if you drink alcohol and take the drug

□ B   This drug has no effect on alcohol

□ C   This drug will make your heart beat faster if you drink alcohol as well

□ D   This drug will make you feel sleepier if you drink alcohol as well

□ E   This drug will make it more difficult to breathe if you drink alcohol as well

30 Mrs G, a 32-year-old patient, has been commenced on ketoconazole 2% cream. She has no known drug allergies. You are about to check Mrs G's prescription and notice that she also takes:

   Apixaban tablets 5 mg BD
   Co-codamol tablets 30/500 mg TWO QDS

   Which of the following is the most appropriate course of action to take?

   ☐ A   Dispense the ketoconazole 2% cream
   ☐ B   Ring the doctor and recommend an alternative medication be prescribed instead of ketoconazole
   ☐ C   Ring the doctor and inform them you are advising the patient to stop taking co-codamol for the duration of treatment with ketoconazole
   ☐ D   Ring the doctor and inform them you are advising the patient to stop taking apixaban for the duration of treatment with ketoconazole
   ☐ E   Dispense the prescription and tell the patient to wear additional protective clothing in the sun

31 Ms Z, a 15-year-old patient, has been commenced on insulin therapy. She currently takes no other medication and has no known drug allergies. She has been told to drink *Lucozade Energy Original* drink when her blood sugar is low. She would like to know how much to drink. Which of the following is the most appropriate response?

   ☐ A   For 10 g of carbohydrate drink 90 mL
   ☐ B   For 10 g of carbohydrate drink 100 mL
   ☐ C   For 10 g of carbohydrate drink 110 mL
   ☐ D   For 10 g of carbohydrate drink 120 mL
   ☐ E   For 10 g of carbohydrate drink 130 mL

32 Ms Y, a 25-year-old woman, has come to the community pharmacy. She would like to speak to the pharmacist about emergency contraception. She currently takes no other medication and has no known drug allergies. She tells you that she has a 3-month old baby whom she is breast-feeding. Unprotected sexual intercourse took place 4 days ago and she is worried about being pregnant. She would like to take something immediately as an emergency contraceptive. Which of the following is the most appropriate response?

   ☐ A   Recommend she takes levonorgesterol immediately
   ☐ B   Recommend she takes two tablets of levonorgesterol: one now and one after the next time she breast-feeds

    ☐ C   Recommend she takes two tablets of ulipristal immediately
    ☐ D   Recommend she takes ulipristal immediately but advise her that she will not be able to breast-feed for 1 week
    ☐ E   Recommend she sees her GP to have an intrauterine contraceptive device fitted

33 Ms Y, a 25-year-old woman, has come to the community pharmacy. She would like to speak to the pharmacist about emergency contraception. She currently takes no other medication and has no known drug allergies. She tells you that she has a 5-month-old baby whom she is breast-feeding. Unprotected sexual intercourse took place 2 days ago and she is worried about being pregnant. She would like to take something immediately as an emergency contraceptive.
Which of the following is the most appropriate response?

    ☐ A   Recommend she takes levonorgesterol immediately
    ☐ B   Recommend she takes two tablets of levonorgesterol: one now and one after the next time she breast-feeds
    ☐ C   Recommend she takes two tablets of ulipristal immediately
    ☐ D   Recommend she takes ulipristal immediately, but advise her that she will not be able to breast-feed for 1 week
    ☐ E   Recommend she sees her GP to have an intrauterine contraceptive device fitted

34 Mr J, a 36-year-old man, has come to the community pharmacy. He would like to speak to the pharmacist about his nails. He currently takes no other medication and has no known drug allergies. He tells you that he thinks he has a fungal nail infection. On closer inspection you see that his thumbnail has become yellow and appears thickened. He would like to purchase something from the pharmacy today to treat this.
Which of the following is the most appropriate course of action to take?

    ☐ A   Recommend he purchases amorolfine 5% nail lacquer
    ☐ B   Recommend he purchases amorolfine 5% nail lacquer and advise that it normally takes 6 months for the infection to be treated
    ☐ C   Recommend he purchases amorolfine 5% nail lacquer and advise that it normally takes 12 months for the infection to be treated
    ☐ D   Recommend he purchases amorolfine 5% nail lacquer and advise that it normally takes 18 months for the infection to be treated
    ☐ E   Refer him to his GP

35 Mrs K, a 30-year-old woman, has come to the community pharmacy. She would like to speak to the pharmacist about her nails. She currently takes an oral contraceptive pill, citalopram 20 mg tablets OD and metformin 500 mg TDS. She has no known drug allergies. She tells you that she thinks she has a fungal nail infection. On closer inspection you see that two of her nails on her left foot have become yellow and appear thickened. She would like to purchase something from the pharmacy today to treat this.
Which of the following is the most appropriate course of action to take?

   ☐ A Recommend she purchases amorolfine 5% nail lacquer from a podiatrist
   ☐ B Recommend she purchases amorolfine 5% nail lacquer and advise that it can take approximately 3 months for the infection to be treated
   ☐ C Recommend she purchases amorolfine 5% nail lacquer and advise that it normally takes 6 months for the infection to be treated
   ☐ D Recommend she purchases amorolfine 5% nail lacquer and advise that it normally takes 9 months for the infection to be treated
   ☐ E Refer her to her GP

36 Mrs A, a 32-year-old woman, has come to the community pharmacy. She would like to speak to the pharmacist about her weight. She currently takes an oral contraceptive pill and levothyroxine tablets. She has no known drug allergies. She tells you that she would like to purchase orlistat 60 mg capsules over the counter. You calculate her BMI to be 30 kg/m².
Which of the following is the most appropriate course of action to take?

   ☐ A Recommend she purchases orlistat 60 mg capsules
   ☐ B Recommend she purchases orlistat 60 mg capsules and discuss adopting a low-fat diet
   ☐ C Recommend she purchases orlistat 60 mg capsules and discuss adopting a low-fat diet that is mildly hypocaloric
   ☐ D Recommend she purchases orlistat 60 mg capsules and uses additional contraceptive measures if she experiences diarrhoea
   ☐ E Refer her to her GP

37 Mrs D, a 22-year-old woman, has come to the community pharmacy. She would like to speak to the pharmacist about her weight. She

currently takes sodium valproate tablets, and has no known drug allergies. She tells you that she would like to purchase orlistat 60 mg capsules over the counter. You calculate her BMI to be 32 kg/m². Which of the following is the most appropriate course of action to take?

☐ A Recommend she purchases orlistat 60 mg capsules
☐ B Recommend she purchases orlistat 60 mg capsules and discuss adopting a low-fat diet
☐ C Recommend she purchases orlistat 60 mg capsules and discuss adopting a low-fat diet that is mildly hypocaloric
☐ D Recommend she purchases orlistat 60 mg capsules and to take two capsules three times daily
☐ E Refer her to her GP

38 Mr J, a 17-year-old man, has come to the community pharmacy. He would like to speak to the pharmacist about his weight. He currently takes no other medication and has no known drug allergies. He tells you that he would like to purchase orlistat 60 mg capsules over the counter. You calculate his BMI to be 34 kg/m². Which of the following is the most appropriate course of action to take?

☐ A Recommend he purchases orlistat 60 mg capsules
☐ B Recommend he purchases orlistat 60 mg capsules and discuss adopting a low-fat diet
☐ C Recommend he purchases orlistat 60 mg capsules and discuss adopting a low-fat diet that is mildly hypocaloric
☐ D Recommend he purchases orlistat 60 mg capsules and to take two capsules three times daily
☐ E Refer him to his GP

39 Mrs T, a 23-year-old woman, has come to the community pharmacy. She would like to speak to the pharmacist about her eye. She currently takes an oral contraceptive pill and levothyroxine tablets. She has no known drug allergies. She tells you that she would like to purchase chloramphenicol 1% eye drops as she thinks she has an eye infection. On questioning you discover that her eye condition has worsened as the rash on her cheek has worsened. Which of the following is the most appropriate course of action to take?

☐ A Recommend she purchases chloramphenicol 1% eye drops
☐ B Recommend she purchases chloramphenicol 1% eye drops and uses them for 5 days

☐ C   Recommend she purchases chloramphenicol 1% eye drops and uses them for 7 days

☐ D   Recommend she purchases chloramphenicol 1% eye drops and uses them for 14 days

☐ E   Refer her to the GP

40   Mr P, a 54-year-old man, has come to the community pharmacy. He would like to speak to the pharmacist about his eye. He currently takes lisinopril 10 mg tablets OD. He has no known drug allergies. He tells you that he would like to purchase chloramphenicol 1% eye drops as he thinks he has an eye infection. On questioning you discover that his eye condition developed after he was cutting wood at the weekend, and felt something go into his eye.

Which of the following is the most appropriate course of action to take?

☐ A   Recommend he purchases chloramphenicol 1% eye drops

☐ B   Recommend he purchases chloramphenicol 1% eye drops and uses them for 5 days

☐ C   Recommend he purchases chloramphenicol 1% eye drops and uses them for 7 days

☐ D   Recommend he purchases chloramphenicol 1% eye drops and uses them for 14 days

☐ E   Refer him to his GP

SECTION D

Oksana Pyzik

1   Which of the following is NOT associated with an increased risk of haemorrhage with dabigatran?

☐ A   moderate renal impairment
☐ B   age (≥75 years)
☐ C   low body weight
☐ D   obesity
☐ E   taken concomitantly with SSRIs

2   Which of the following is a risk factor for developing acute pyelonephritis?

☐ A   kidney stones
☐ B   heart failure
☐ C   hypertension
☐ D   hypercholesterolaemia
☐ E   obesity

3   Which of the following pathogens is most commonly indicated in cradle cap?

☐ A   *Helicobacter pylori*
☐ B   *Streptococcus pyogenes*
☐ C   *Malassezia* spp.
☐ D   *Mycobacterium* spp.
☐ E   *Yersinia pestis*

4   Which of the following medicines is indicated for the treatment of androgenic alopecia?

☐ A   finasteride 1 mg tablets
☐ B   dutasteride 500 mcg tablets
☐ C   tadalafil 20 mg tablets
☐ D   tamsulosin 400 mcg tablets
☐ E   minoxidil 5 mg tablets

5   A 25-year-old woman who suffers from epilepsy is trying to get pregnant.

What dose of folic acid should she be prescribed?

   ☐ A   1000 mcg
   ☐ B   400 mcg
   ☐ C   40 mg
   ☐ D   20 mg
   ☐ E   5 mg

6   A patient with which one of the following conditions may buy sildenafil over the counter?

   ☐ A   unstable angina
   ☐ B   hypotension
   ☐ C   recent myocardial infarction
   ☐ D   recent stroke
   ☐ E   high cholesterol

7   Which of the following statements concerning the withdrawal of anti-epileptic therapy is correct?

   ☐ A   Withdraw anti-epileptic drugs gradually over a period of 4–6 weeks
   ☐ B   Withdraw benzodiazepines over a period of 2–3 months
   ☐ C   The decision to withdraw should be taken primarily by the specialist
   ☐ D   The patient must be seizure-free for at least 5 years
   ☐ E   Withdraw one drug at a time if on multiple regimes

8   Mr TM appears at the pharmacy asking for your advice. He has developed hypopigmented macules and patches on his left arm and upper back. The patches started small but have coalesced together, and now cover the entire back of his arm and upper back. He is self-conscious about the discoloration and has been wearing long sleeves to hide the patches. You examine the skin and notice the patches to be slightly pink in colour and covered in a fine powdery scale. Upon further questioning, you discover that the patches are not painful and he does not have these patches anywhere else.
Which of the following conditions is Mr TM most likely to be suffering from?

   ☐ A   eczema
   ☐ B   psoriasis
   ☐ C   pityriasis versicolor
   ☐ D   rosacea
   ☐ E   vitiligo

9   Which of the following is LEAST likely to be associated with oropharyngeal cancer?

   ☐ A   Infection with human papillomavirus (HPV)
   ☐ B   A history of smoking for more than 10 years
   ☐ C   Infection with herpes simplex virus
   ☐ D   Chewing betel – a stimulant liquid commonly used in South America
   ☐ E   Drinking maté – a stimulant liquid commonly used in parts of Asia

10 Mr LW is a 32-year-old man who presents at your pharmacy with a fever, headache, fatigue, severe joint pain, swollen knees and a skin rash on his back. On questioning the patient you discover that the rash has expanded gradually over the past few days from 12 cm to 30 cm, and is circular in appearance, resembling a target or 'bull's eye'. He explains that he is an avid hiker and 1 month ago he spent his holiday camping in the New Forest. He recalls that there were many mosquitoes in the forest.
   Which of the following conditions is Mr LW most likely to have?

   ☐ A   lyme disease
   ☐ B   malaria
   ☐ C   ringworm
   ☐ D   southern tick-associated rash illness (STARI)
   ☐ E   urticaria multiforme

11 Which of the following symptoms is NOT a sign of vitamin B_{12} deficiency?

   ☐ A   ataxia
   ☐ B   erythematous rash
   ☐ C   glossitis
   ☐ D   paraesthesia
   ☐ E   visual disturbance

12 Which of the following is not linked as a causal agent of macrocytosis?

   ☐ A   anti-neoplastic medicines
   ☐ B   excessive alcohol intake
   ☐ C   non-steroidal anti-inflammatory medicines
   ☐ D   vitamin B_{12} deficiency
   ☐ E   liver disease

13 Which of the following drug combinations is known to have an increased risk of myopathy?

 ☐ A ibuprofen with paracetamol
 ☐ B digoxin with amiodarone
 ☐ C beclometasone with theophylline
 ☐ D simvastatin with gemfibrozil
 ☐ E phenytoin with atenolol

14 Which of the following types of melanoma is the most common in the UK?

 ☐ A acral lentiginous melanoma
 ☐ B amelanotic melanoma
 ☐ C lentigo maligna melanoma
 ☐ D nodular melanoma
 ☐ E superficial spreading melanoma

15 A 34-year-old woman who is taking carbimazole for the treatment of thyrotoxicosis complains of a sore throat.
Which of the following tests would be most important to do in this case?

 ☐ A blood cultures
 ☐ B C-reactive protein
 ☐ C neutrophil count
 ☐ D throat swab
 ☐ E thyroid function test

16 A 42-year-old man develops a rash with small red spots all over his body. On further questioning, you discover that the rash is intensely itchy and worse at night, and you see that he has wavy, silver-coloured lines on his skin.
Which one of the following diagnoses is most likely?

 ☐ A acne
 ☐ B eczema
 ☐ C chickenpox
 ☐ D hives
 ☐ E scabies

17 Which one of the following is the LEAST appropriate advice to give a patient suffering from vaginal thrush?

 ☐ A Apply external cream thinly to the vulva and labia two to three times a day

☐ B   Insert the 500 mg pessary high into the vagina in the morning

☐ C   You may experience pelvic or abdominal pain or vaginal bleeding after using the pessary

☐ D   Avoid cleaning the vulval area more than once a day

☐ E   Do not use the pessary during your menstrual cycle

18   A 58-year-old man has suffered from several attacks of gout over the last 3 months. He had a heart attack 2 years ago and is diabetic. His prescriber starts him on allopurinol to prevent gout.
Which of the following statements with regard to his treatment is correct?

☐ A   Allopurinol is used to treat acute gout

☐ B   Start allopurinol 4–6 weeks after the inflammation has settled, because the drug may precipitate further attacks

☐ C   Take a low dose of an NSAID or colchicine with allopurinol for 1 month

☐ D   A urinary output of not less than 1 litre a day must be maintained in all patients receiving allopurinol

☐ E   Check the serum uric acid (SUA) level and renal function at 6 months

19   Which of the following statements is LEAST aligned with the principles of prescribing treatments for infectious diseases?

☐ A   Limit prescribing over the telephone to exceptional cases

☐ B   Consider giving a delayed prescription for an upper respiratory tract infection

☐ C   Avoid the widespread use of topical antibiotics

☐ D   Avoid narrow-spectrum antibiotics where broad-spectrum antibiotics remain effective

☐ E   In pregnancy, take specimens to inform treatment and, where possible, avoid tetracyclines, aminoglycosides and quinolones

20   A newborn at 8 weeks is given a vaccine via the oral route.
Which of the following vaccines did the child receive?

☐ A   Bacille Calmette–Guérin (BCG) vaccine

☐ B   diphtheria, tetanus and pertussis (DTaP) vaccine

☐ C   hepatitis B vaccine

☐ D   human papillomavirus (HPV) vaccine

☐ E   rotavirus vaccine

For questions 21–23 refer to the following extract: https://www.medicines
.org.uk/emc/medicine/11363

21 A-65-year-old man has been prescribed tadalafil 5 mg tablets. He has
type 2 diabetes and his last blood pressure reading was 130/90 mmHg.
He is retired and leads a sedentary lifestyle, despite his doctor's recommendation to increase his level of physical activity. Lately he has been
complaining of increased frequency of urination at night. He has done
some research online about this medicine because he has not taken it
before. He presents at the pharmacy with his wife to ask you some
questions about this treatment because he is confused by the conflicting
information he has read online.
Which of the following statements is true?

☐ A   He is being treated for erectile dysfunction
☐ B   He should refrain from drinking alcohol
☐ C   He is elderly and therefore a dose adjustment is required
☐ D   He has diabetes and therefore the dose should be increased
☐ E   He may experience a transient decrease in blood pressure

22 After a check-up with his GP he has been prescribed an additional
medicine.
Which of the following medicines is contraindicated when taken
together with tadalafil?

☐ A   aspirin
☐ B   dabigatran
☐ C   glyceryl trinitrate
☐ D   ramipril
☐ E   warfarin

23 His prescriber has discontinued his tadalafil treatment.
Which of the following conditions would NOT be a reason for discon-
tinuing treatment with tadalafil?

☐ A   Myocardial infarction within the last 90 days
☐ B   Cerebrovascular accident in the last 6 months
☐ C   Uncontrolled arrhythmias
☐ D   Unstable angina
☐ E   Hypertension

24 A 53-year-old woman with breast cancer has had a total mastec-
tomy. She has been prescribed tamoxifen 20 mg for positive oestrogen
receptors on the tumour.

Which of the following counselling points is the correct advice to give?

- [ ] A Tamoxifen reduces the risk of endometrial cancer
- [ ] B Tamoxifen interacts with warfarin because it reduces its efficacy
- [ ] C Take at night to reduce symptoms of hot flushes
- [ ] D Take once weekly
- [ ] E Report to hospital immediately if there is any redness, pain or swelling of the legs

25 A 85-year-old man is receiving palliative care for pancreatic cancer and has been prescribed *Zomorph* 200 mg capsules BD to relieve pain. He is immobile, has had trouble eating and drinking, and is slightly dehydrated.
Which of the following medicines may predispose to faecal impaction in this patient?

- [ ] A co-danthramer
- [ ] B diclofenac
- [ ] C ispaghula husk
- [ ] D ketamine
- [ ] E lactulose

26 A 29-year-old woman who is in the third trimester of pregnancy seeks your advice about receiving the flu vaccine.
Which of the following statements is correct with regard to administration of the flu vaccine in pregnant women?

- [ ] A Pregnant women are more likely to suffer side-effects from the influenza vaccine
- [ ] B The influenza vaccine is contraindicated in the first trimester of pregnancy
- [ ] C The influenza vaccine is contraindicated in the third trimester of pregnancy
- [ ] D Pregnant women who have received an influenza vaccine are at slightly more risk of miscarriage
- [ ] E An influenza vaccine given to the mother may provide passive immunity to the infant in the first few months of life

27 A 35-year-old woman travelled to Brazil for a 2-week holiday in August. On her return she presents with symptoms of conjunctivitis and a rash. She is worried due to the outbreak of Zika in the area and she is trying to get pregnant. Her partner remained in the UK and presents with no symptoms.

Which of the following is the shortest amount of time that is considered safe to conceive after travel to areas with active Zika transmission?

☐ A 8 weeks
☐ B 12 weeks
☐ C 6 months
☐ D 9 months
☐ E 12 months

28 A 52-year-old woman with hypertension and bipolar disorder is admitted into hospital due to a seizure, which she experienced for the first time. According to the SCR, there have been no recent dose changes of lithium. Her moods have been stable; however, the patient complains of constant fatigue. You note from the SCR that she was recently prescribed bendroflumethiazide and enalapril.
You request the following tests:

	Value	Normal range
Urea (mmol/L)	5	3–7
Cr (mmol/L)	144	60–125
Na (mmol/L)	140	133–145
K (mmol/L)	4.0	3.5–5.0
Li (mmol/L)	2.2	0.4–0.8

Which of the following changes would you recommend?

☐ A Increase the dose of lithium and decrease the dose of enalapril
☐ B Stop lithium and stop enalapril
☐ C Decrease the dose of lithium and stop bendroflumethiazide
☐ D Stop lithium and stop bendroflumethiazide
☐ E Stop lithium, stop bendroflumethiazide and stop enalapril

29 A 33-year-old man presents with red, itchy, watery eyes and symptoms of general malaise. You suspect that he may be suffering from viral conjunctivitis.
What pathogen is responsible for most cases of viral conjunctivitis?

☐ A adenovirus
☐ B Epstein–Barr virus
☐ C Norwalk virus
☐ D rhinovirus
☐ E rotavirus

30 A 75-year-old patient is diagnosed with congestive heart failure. He also suffers from type 2 diabetes and has mild hypertension. He suffered a mild stroke last year as a result of non-valvular atrial fibrillation. Which of the following anticoagulants would be most appropriate for this patient?

- [ ] A acenocoumarol
- [ ] B apixaban
- [ ] C aspirin
- [ ] D phenindione
- [ ] E warfarin

31 A 74-year-old patient presents with anal itching and bright red, painless, rectal bleeding. He has been diagnosed with haemorrhoids and has been prescribed a cream that contains hydrocortisone. Which of the following would you dispense to this patient?

- [ ] A *Anacal*
- [ ] B *Anusol*
- [ ] C *Anodesyn*
- [ ] D *Germoloids*
- [ ] E *Proctosedyl*

32 Which of the following statements correctly describes a grade 4 haemorrhoid?

- [ ] A Large with permanent prolapse from within the anus
- [ ] B Prolapse from the anus triggered by defecation
- [ ] C Partial prolapse triggered by defecation
- [ ] D Small swellings on the inside of the anal canal
- [ ] E Small swellings that cannot be seen or felt from outside the anus

33 A 70-year-old man is brought to the accident and emergency department by his carer because she noticed that there was blood in his urine. He is currently taking warfarin for atrial fibrillation. In hospital his INR reaches 8.2. Within which of the following ranges should his INR fall?

- [ ] A 1.0
- [ ] B 2.5
- [ ] C 3.5
- [ ] D 4.0
- [ ] E 5.0

34 A 52-year-old man who has Parkinson's disease has been prescribed a catechol-O-methyltransferase (COMT) inhibitor. He asks to speak with the pharmacist about the reports of fatal liver toxicity associated with this drug.
Which of the following medicines has been prescribed for this patient?

- ☐ **A** cabergoline
- ☐ **B** entacapone
- ☐ **C** rasagiline
- ☐ **D** selegiline
- ☐ **E** tolcapone

35 Mrs AS, a 66-year-old woman who has deep vein thrombosis, has suffered a minor stroke and been admitted to hospital. Her records indicate a history of breast cancer, cluster headaches and type 2 diabetes.
Which of her following medicines should be discontinued?

- ☐ **A** enoxaparin
- ☐ **B** insulin
- ☐ **C** metformin
- ☐ **D** sitagliptin
- ☐ **E** verapamil

36 A 58-year-old man who is suffering from lung cancer is undergoing treatment with vincristine. He starts to feel a painful stinging sensation at the injection site which you suspect indicates that the drug is being extravasated.
What action should NOT be taken in this situation?

- ☐ **A** Apply a hot pack
- ☐ **B** Elevate limb
- ☐ **C** Administer hyaluronidase
- ☐ **D** Aspirate through the cannula to remove as much of the residual drug as possible
- ☐ **E** Stop IV infusion immediately

37 A 24-year-old woman presents with the following symptoms: weight loss, sensitivity to heat, anxiety, trembling, tachycardia and waking throughout the night due to stress.
Which of the following medicines may be contributing to these symptoms?

- ☐ **A** azithromycin 1 g
- ☐ **B** citalopram 10 mg

☐ C levothyroxine 125 mcg
☐ D *Microgynon 30*
☐ E sulfasalazine 1 g

38 With regard to the measles, mumps and rubella (MMR) vaccine, which of the following counselling points is correct?

☐ A Every child should receive one dose of MMR vaccine before entry to primary school, unless there is a valid contraindication

☐ B MMR vaccine may also be used in the control of outbreaks of measles and should be offered to susceptible children aged >2 months who are contacts of a case, within 3 days of exposure to infection

☐ C It should be administered to children at 4 months of age.

☐ D A booster shot should be given 10 years later

☐ E MMR vaccine is not suitable for prophylaxis after exposure to mumps or rubella

39 A 36-year-old woman presents at the pharmacy requesting an ovulation prediction kit.
The test kit will measure the concentration in the urine of which of the following hormones?

☐ A follicle-stimulating hormone (FSH)
☐ B human chorionic gonadotrophin
☐ C luteinising hormone (LH)
☐ D oestrogen
☐ E progesterone

40 A 5-year-old boy presents with pyrexia, nausea and vomiting, a painful right hand and a non-blanching rash that appeared yesterday. The child has no history of trauma but is reluctant to be touched. The parents administered paracetamol 3 hours ago; however, his temperature remains at 39.9°C.
Which of the following diagnoses is correct?

☐ A chickenpox
☐ B measles
☐ C meningitis
☐ D mumps
☐ E rubella

Extended matching
questions

Ryan Hamilton

In this section, for each numbered question, select the one lettered option that most closely corresponds to the answer. Within each group of questions each lettered option may be used once, more than once or not at all.

Antibacterials

A   amoxicillin
B   clarithromycin
C   lymecycline
D   metronidazole
E   nitrofurantoin
F   rifampicin
G   trimethoprim
H   vancomycin

For questions 1–6

For the patients described below, select the single most likely antibacterial agent from the list above. Each option may be used once, more than once or not at all.

1   Mrs Y has been prescribed two antibacterial agents to treat an infection on her prosthetic knee implant. She comes into your pharmacy to collect the next instalment of her treatment and mentions that her urine has

recently been a dark reddish colour. You advise her that one of her antibiotics is causing this and is generally harmless.

2   Mrs U has been diagnosed with a lower urinary tract infection, caused by a fully sensitive strain of *E. coli*. However, she should not be prescribed this usual first-line agent because her glomerular filtration rate is only 41 mL/min and taking this medicine risks treatment failure.

3   Mr S has just been diagnosed with a mild *C. difficile* infection after taking antibiotics for cellulitis. Mr S has not had *C. difficile* diarrhoea before so his GP decides to prescribe the first-line choice antibiotic to treat this new infection.

4   Mrs F has been admitted to your acute medical unit with severe diarrhoea, which the medical team believe is secondary to repeated treatments for urinary tract infections. She is diagnosed with severe *C. difficile* infection and is prescribed intravenous treatment. However, you explain that the prescribed antibiotic must not be given intravenously for *C. difficile* infection as it does not penetrate into the bowel and so will not treat the infection.

5   The medical team have prescribed an intravenous infusion for a patient, Mr B, who requires treatment for cellulitis. On checking the prescription you note that the prescribed rate of infusion is too quick, so you advise the nurse to give it at a slower rate to avoid a group of adverse reactions commonly known as 'red man' or 'red neck' syndrome.

6   Miss K has been suffering from a chest infection for over a week, which her GP has tried to treat with first-line antibiotics. However, Miss K's condition does not improve and her GP diagnoses her with probable community-acquired pneumonia, of increasing severity. Her GP discusses treatment options with you and you suggest he add in a second antibacterial agent that will cover atypical pathogens.

Diabetes mellitus

A   *Actrapid* (insulin soluble human)
B   canagliflozin
C   exenatide
D   glibenclamide
E   gliclazide
F   *Humalog Mix25*® (biphasic insulin lispro)
G   *Lantus* (insulin glargine)
H   linagliptin
I   metformin

For questions 7–10

For the patients described below, select the single most likely medicine from the list above. Each option may be used once, more than once or not at all.

7 Mr J has been admitted to hospital with shortness of breath and has been diagnosed with an acute episode of heart failure. After taking his drug history you advise the medical team to withhold this medicine as it can increase the risk of Mr J developing lactic acidosis.

8 Mr U, who is 18 years old, is admitted to your high-dependency unit with diabetic ketoacidosis. In order to drive down his serum glucose and ketones, the medical team prescribe a continuous intravenous infusion of this medicine.

9 Mrs E comes into your pharmacy with her regular prescription. Whilst it is being dispensed she asks you whether she should drink more cranberry juice, or anything else you would advise, to prevent urinary tract infections. On further questioning, you find she has recently been treated for two such infections and you advise that she speaks to her GP as one of her diabetes medicines can increase her risk of developing urinary tract infections.

10 Mr X has been taking medicines for type 2 diabetes for 10 years but has recently lost control of his HbA1c and was started on a new medicine. However, a few weeks later he complains of tiredness and dizzy spells, which he associated with low blood sugar levels. You note that his new medicine does not cause hypoglycaemic episodes on its own, but can increase the risk of hypoglycaemia when added to other diabetes medicines.

Respiratory medicines

A beclometasone
B montelukast
C omalizumab
D salbutamol
E salmeterol
F sodium chloride 7%
G theophylline
H tiotropium

For questions 11–16

For the patients described below, select the single most likely medicine from the list above. Each option may be used once, more than once or not at all.

11 This medicine should be used in combination with another medicine in patients with COPD as the combination has been found to be effective in treating COPD and using this medicine alone can increase the risk of respiratory tract infections.

12 Miss S has been admitted to hospital with a severe exacerbation of asthma and requires nebulised therapy. You advise that one of the medicines can be given as a continuous nebulisation if necessary.

13 Mr R has been prescribed an inhaler for newly diagnosed asthma. You explain that when he has taken this medicine he should rinse his mouth to prevent the development of oral infections such as thrush.

14 Mrs T is well known to you and she comes into your pharmacy to collect her COPD medicines. You note that she looks restless and agitated so you ask her if she is okay. She mentions that she has been feeling nauseated for the past few days and that her heart feels like it is racing. You advise Mrs T to visit the urgent care centre today as you think it may be one of her medicines that is causing these symptoms.

15 Mr N, an 84-year-old man who is well known to your pharmacy, has been taking medicines for COPD for the past 20 years but has recently been diagnosed with renal impairment. You check his SCR and note his renal function (eGFR) is only $37\,\mathrm{mL/min}$ per $1.73\,\mathrm{m^2}$. You call his GP to discuss one of his medicines, as you think an alternative may be more appropriate.

16 Mrs M has been admitted to your respiratory ward with a severe exacerbation of COPD, for which she is being treated with nebulised and intravenous therapies. You advise the respiratory physicians to monitor serum concentrations of one of these medicines to ensure treatment is within the desired range.

Medicines used in epilepsy

A   carbamazepine
B   gabapentin
C   lamotrigine
D   levetiracetam

E midazolam
F phenytoin
G sodium valproate
H topiramate

For questions 17–20

For the patients described below, select the single most likely medicine from the list above. Each option may be used once, more than once or not at all.

17 Adam is a 4-year-old boy who has been diagnosed with epilepsy and has been prescribed a medicine that should be used when he has a seizure. You decide to sit down with his parents and teach them now to give this medicine, which needs to be given via the buccal route.

18 Mrs L has been admitted to your ward suffering from blurred vision, ataxia, dizziness and drowsiness. On reconciliation of her medicines you find that she has recently been prescribed clarithromycin for a respiratory tract infection, which you believe is interacting with one of her epilepsy medicines and causing the symptoms that resulted in her admission to hospital.

19 Mr A has been taken to the emergency department with sepsis secondary to a possible respiratory tract infection, for which he is given a dose of meropenem. The next day Mr A experiences a seizure, which the medical team believe is due to his infection and sepsis. However, you also warn the medical team that meropenem can interact with one of Mr A's epilepsy medicines, leading to greatly depleted serum concentrations.

20 Miss T comes into your pharmacy and asks to speak to you in private. She has recently moved in with her partner and is thinking about having a baby. She seeks your advice as you know her and her medicines well. You note that one of her medicines, which she takes for epilepsy, could increase the risk of malformations and neural tube defects. You supply her with folic acid supplements and advise her to see her GP as soon as possible.

Antihypertensive medicines

A amlodipine
B bendroflumethiazide
C bisoprolol

D   hydralazine
E   losartan
F   moxonidine
G   ramipril
H   verapamil

For questions 21–23

For the patients described below, select the single most likely medicine from the list above. Each option may be used once, more than once or not at all.

21   Mr Y has worsening hypertension and his GP has decided to add in another agent to his treatment. However, on presenting you with his prescription you note that there is a potentially serious interaction between this new medicine and his current beta-blocker therapy, which could result in heart block.

22   Mrs S comes into the pharmacy where you are the locum to collect her medicines. She has been taking a number of medicines since suffering from a heart attack 2 months ago. Whilst talking to her she mentions that she has been feeling short of breath, tight chested at night and more tired than usual. You check her PMR and see a number of inhalers, which you confirm are for asthma. You advise Mrs S to speak to her GP as you believe one of her medicines may be exacerbating her asthma.

23   Mr H comes into your pharmacy to collect a short course of colchicine for acute gout. Whilst checking his PMR you notice that one of his medicines may have precipitated gout and you decide to call Mr H's GP to discuss this.

Laxatives

A   arachis oil
B   bisacodyl
C   docusate sodium
D   ispaghula husk
E   lactulose
F   macrogols
G   methylnaltrexone
H   prucalopride
I   senna

For questions 24–28

For the patients described below, select the single most likely medicine from the list above. Each option may be used once, more than once or not at all.

24 Mrs O has been suffering from ongoing constipation as a result of using fentanyl patches. After trying a number of laxative agents alone, and in combination, her medical team asks you for advice. You suggest that the constipation is due to opioid activity in the gut and suggest a drug that has antagonistic action on these receptors.

25 Mr U comes into your pharmacy as he has been suffering from constipation over the past week but can't get an appointment at the doctor for another week. You find that he is lactose intolerant, so advise him against taking one of the laxatives that is available over the counter.

26 Mr W has been admitted to your ward with faecal impaction, which is later found to be secondary to colonic atony. You review his drug chart and decide to cross off a medicine because it is contraindicated in this circumstance.

27 One of the nurses on your ward asks you for advice about a laxative that has been prescribed for one of her patients. You tell her that she should not give this laxative to this patient as the patient is allergic to peanuts.

28 Mr G, an elderly man on your ward, has been prescribed an osmotic and a stimulant laxative for the past week, but this has not helped his constipation. On discussing other oral options with the medical team, you suggest that a different laxative could be tried as it acts as a wetting agent to soften stools.

Immunomodulatory medicines

A azathioprine
B basiliximab
C ciclosporin
D fingolimod
E methotrexate
F mycophenolate
G prednisolone
H tacrolimus

For questions 29 and 30

For the patients described below, select the single most likely medicine from the list above. Each option may be used once, more than once or not at all.

29 Mr Q has been started on this medicine to prevent rejection of his transplanted kidney. Whilst counselling Mr Q on this new medicine, you advise him that it could affect his ability to drive or perform skilled tasks.

30 Mrs F presents you with a prescription for a new medicine for worsening Crohn's disease. You decide to call her GP because she should also be taking folic acid on a different day to this medicine.

Counselling points

A Dissolve or mix with water before taking
B Do not drink alcohol
C Do not take milk, indigestion remedies or medicines containing iron or zinc 2 hours before or after you take this medicine
D Doses should be taken with plenty of water while sitting or standing, on an empty stomach at least 30 minutes before breakfast
E Protect your skin from sunlight – even on a bright but cloudy day. Do not use sunbeds
F Take 30–60 minutes before food
G Take with or just after food, or a meal
H This medicine may make you sleepy

For questions 31–36

For the patients described below, select the single most likely counselling point from the list above. Each option may be used once, more than once or not at all.

31 Mrs A has been newly started on amiodarone by the cardiology consultant. When reviewing her discharge prescription you decide to talk to her and give her some important information about this medicine.

32 Mrs P presents you with a new prescription for alendronic acid, 70 mg once a week.

33 Mr U has been suffering from ongoing heartburn, for which you refer him to his GP. The next week he comes to your pharmacy with a prescription for lansoprazole capsules, 15 mg once daily.

34 Miss C comes into your pharmacy for her annual MUR. While discussing her medicines and general lifestyle, you find that her blood sugars are not as well controlled as they used to be. You decide to provide her with some information about her metformin.

35 Mr F presents to your outpatient pharmacy with a prescription for ciprofloxacin, which he needs to take for 7 days for a urinary tract infection. When giving out the prescription you confirm he has not taken this medicine before and decide to give him some specific counselling.

36 George, a 7-year-old boy, has been newly diagnosed with epilepsy and his neurologist has started him on sodium valproate modified-release tablets. When handing this medicine over to his mum you decide to give her, and George, some information about this medicine.

Research and evaluation

A   audit
B   case–control study
C   focus group
D   meta-analysis
E   open label study
F   PDSA cycle
G   quality improvement project
H   randomised control trial
I   root cause analysis

For questions 37–40

For the scenarios described below, select the single most likely research and evaluation method from the list above. Each option may be used once, more than once or not at all.

37 This is considered the highest level of evidence that can be used to develop clinical guidelines.

38 You are a community pharmacist and you want to ensure that cough medicines are being supplied appropriately OTC. You design a small project to collect information on which products are being supplied for which indications, from which you aim to identify any improvements or interventions that you can make.

39 You are working on a respiratory ward and undertake a study that shows that the aminophylline infusion chart is not being followed correctly. You design a short project whereby you will introduce an updated aminophylline chart, measure the impact of this new chart and identify any further actions needed.

40 A patient on your ward has come to serious harm from a medicine. You decide to investigate how this error could have occurred to ensure that processes and barriers can be put in place to prevent the same error from happening again

SECTION B

Simon Harris

In this section, for each numbered question, select the one lettered option that most closely corresponds to the answer. Within each group of questions each lettered option may be used once, more than once or not at all.

Vaccination intervals

A 8 weeks
B 12 weeks
C 16 weeks
D 12 months
E 5 years
F 18 years
G 45 years
H 70 years

For questions 1–4

For the questions described below, select the most suitable vaccination interval from the list above. Each option may be used once, more than once or not at all.

1 The 5-in-1 vaccine contains diphtheria with *Haemophilus influenzae* type b (Hib) vaccine, pertussis, poliomyelitis and tetanus. At what age would a child born in the UK have their first dose of the 5-in-1 vaccine?

2 From what age is the varicella-zoster vaccine recommended, for the prevention of herpes zoster?

3 At what age is the first dose of the measles, mumps and rubella vaccine administered?

4 At what age is the third dose of tetanus administered to a child as part of the routine immunisation schedule?

Adverse drug reactions

    A   binge eating
    B   confusion
    C   dental pain
    D   hyperglycaemia
    E   mouth ulcers
    F   oily stools
    G   pain in both knees
    H   sweating

For questions 5–7

For the scenarios described below, select the most likely adverse drug reaction from the list above. Each option may be used once, more than once or not at all.

5   A 19-year-old woman has been prescribed trimethoprim 100 mg tablets long term for prophylaxis of recurrent urinary tract infection. Which warning sign should she look out for and report immediately due to the risk of blood disorders?

6   A 63-year-old man is receiving treatment for osteoporosis with zoledronic acid. Which adverse drug reaction should he be reminded to look out for?

7   Which warning sign indicates that a patient on apomorphine should have the drug withdrawn or the dose reduced until the symptoms resolve?

Laxatives

    A   bisacodyl tablets
    B   co-danthramer capsules
    C   *Dioralyte* oral rehydration sachets
    D   docusate sodium capsules
    E   liquid paraffin
    F   *Movicol* oral powder
    G   senna tablets
    H   sterculia sachets

For questions 8 and 9

For the scenarios described below, select the most suitable laxative from the list above. Each option may be used once, more than once or not at all.

8 A patient has asked you for something to relieve constipation. The laxative you offer works by increasing the amount of water in the large bowel.

9 A 31-year-old woman is 16 weeks' pregnant and is suffering from constipation, despite following the suggested lifestyle and dietary changes. You suggest the next recommended course of action.

Antibacterials

A amoxicillin
B azithromycin
C ciprofloxacin
D clindamycin
E flucloxacillin
F fusidic acid
G metronidazole
H tetracycline

For questions 10–13

For the scenarios described below, select the most appropriate antibacterial from the list above. Each option may be used once, more than once or not at all.

10 Cholestatic jaundice and hepatitis may occur very rarely with this medicine, possibly up to 2 months after it has been stopped.

11 The most appropriate oral treatment for a patient with a first episode of mild-to-moderate C. *difficile* infection.

12 The most appropriate treatment as a single dose for a female patient with a non-specific genital infection.

13 This should be used with caution in patients with conditions that predispose to seizures.

Cardiovascular medicines

A   amiodarone
B   bisoprolol
C   dipyridamole
D   furosemide
E   indapamide
F   labetalol
G   nicorandil
H   warfarin

For questions 14–18

For the scenarios described below, select the most appropriate cardio-vascular medicine from the list above. Each option may be used once, more than once or not at all.

14   A 61-year-old woman requires the addition of a new medicine which, once initiated, will require the dose of her simvastatin 40 mg to be reduced.

15   Miss W is a 69-year-old woman with end-stage renal disease, who was admitted to hospital suffering from a painful skin rash. She is wondering if it could be an adverse reaction to one of her medicines.

16   Mr T is a 51-year-old man who is currently taking ramipril 5 mg capsules and amlodipine 10 mg tablets. He checks his blood pressure daily and recently noticed it is no longer controlled. He visits his GP who steps up his treatment and prescribes an additional antihypertensive drug.

17   Miss F is 9.5 weeks' pregnant and, after taking several blood pressure readings, her GP notes that her average blood pressure is 165/100 mmHg. The GP agrees with the patient to begin an antihypertensive drug that is widely used for treating hypertension in pregnancy.

18   Mrs B has stable heart failure due to left ventricular systolic dysfunction and is taking enalapril 20 mg and one other medication, which she has been very slowly increasing the dose of over the past 2 weeks. She has been instructed to continue increasing the dose provided that she continues to tolerate the medicine well.

Endocrine medicines

    A   buserelin
    B   carbimazole
    C   ibandronic acid
    D   liraglutide
    E   norethisterone
    F   prednisolone
    G   propylthiouracil
    H   tibolone

> **For questions 19–21**
>
> For the scenarios described below, select the most appropriate endocrine related medicine from the list above. Each option may be used once, more than once or not at all.

19 Miss M has come to your pharmacy to purchase an over-the-counter remedy for mouth ulcers. You remember she also came into the pharmacy 2 days ago feeling very tired and asking for lozenges for a sore throat. You ask if she is taking any medication, and one of the medicines she lists causes you concern. You advise her to tell her GP immediately about her symptoms.

20 You are delivering a training session for your medicines counter assistants, and explain to them it's vital they report specific symptoms that can be associated with serious adverse drug reactions. You list the symptoms of abdominal pain, yellow and/or itchy skin, and dark urine, and ask them to tell you which medicine these symptoms would cause concern.

21 On dispensing this medicine to a new patient, you advise them to report signs and symptoms of acute pancreatitis such as persistent, severe abdominal pain.

Therapeutic drug monitoring

    A   carbamazepine
    B   digoxin
    C   lithium
    D   phenytoin
    E   tacrolimus
    F   theophylline
    G   valproate
    H   vancomycin

For questions 22–24

For the scenarios described below, select from the list above the drug that is most likely being referred to. Each option may be used once, more than once or not at all.

22   Samples of this drug should be taken 12 hours after the dose to give a serum concentration of 0.4–1.0 mmol/L. Toxicity is made worse by sodium depletion, therefore concurrent use of diuretics should be avoided.

23   For most patients, a plasma concentration of 10–20 mg/L is required, although lower concentrations may be effective. Prescribers and those responsible for the patient should note that plasma concentrations are decreased in smokers and by alcohol consumption.

24   All patients require plasma measurement when receiving this drug, as well as monitoring of auditory function in elderly patients. With IV use, a pre-dose concentration should be around 10–15 mg/L.

Drug interactions

    A   bleeding risk increased
    B   bradycardia
    C   drowsiness
    D   hypertensive crisis
    E   myopathy
    F   Q–T interval prolongation
    G   reduced eGFR
    H   thrombosis

For questions 25 and 26

For the patients described below, select the most likely possible consequence of the drug interaction from the list above. Each option may be used once, more than once or not at all.

25   An 81-year-old man with heart failure has been taking digoxin 125 mcg daily for the past 4 years. He has today been prescribed bisoprolol 1.25 mg daily as an adjunct.

26 A 61-year-old woman has recently been diagnosed with schizophrenia and has been initiated on quetiapine 25 mg twice daily. She also takes amiodarone 200 mg daily.

Electrolyte abnormalities

A hyperglycaemia
B hyperkalaemia
C hypermagnesaemia
D hyperthyroidism
E hypocalcaemia
F hypoglycaemia
G hypokalaemia
H hyponatraemia

For questions 27–30

For the patients described below, select, from the list above, the single most likely drug-induced cause of the patient's symptoms.

27 Mr H is 78 years old and is taking amiodarone 200 mg tablets once daily. For the past few days he has been having palpitations, increased sweating and a feeling of irritability.

28 Mrs L is 35 years old and suffers from tonic–clonic seizures, for which she takes sodium valproate tablets. She brings in her repeat prescription today and tells you she has been feeling confused and restless recently, and doesn't seem to have as much energy as she used to.

29 Mr V is 42 years old and takes perindopril 10 mg each day. He has come to your pharmacy today with a new prescription for spironolactone 25 mg once daily. Before dispensing, you decide to contact Mr V's GP regarding additional monitoring that may be required when taking these two medicines.

30 Whilst working on a hospital ward, you check the drug history of one of your patients and notice they are taking digoxin 125 mcg daily as well as indapamide 2.5 mg daily. You decide to check their recent blood test result as you are concerned about an effect on the levels of one of their electrolytes.

SECTION C

In this section, for each numbered question, select the one lettered option that most closely corresponds to the answer. Within each group of questions each lettered option may be used once, more than once or not at all.

Side-effects

    A   arrhythmia
    B   candidiasis
    C   dry mouth
    D   fine tremor
    E   haematuria
    F   hyperkinesia
    G   sudden onset of sleep
    H   weight loss

For questions 1–8

For the patients described below, select the single most likely side-effect from the list above. Each option may be used once, more than once or not at all.

1   A 34-year-old man who has been initiated on fluticasone propionate 500 mcg, two puffs BD, 4 days ago.

2   A 17-year-old young woman who has been initiated on salbutamol 100 mcg, two puffs QDS PRN, 5 days ago.

3   A 52-year-old woman who has been initiated on tiotropium 18 mcg OD, 7 days ago.

4   A 45-year-old woman who has been initiated on theophylline 250-mg MR capsules OD, 3 days ago.

5   A 3-year-old boy who has been initiated on montelukast 4 mg OD 4 days ago.

6   A 23-year-old woman who has been initiated on roflumilast 500 mcg OD, 3 days ago.

7   A 64-year-old man who has been initiated on cabergoline 1 mg daily, 3 days ago.

8   A 48-year-old woman who has been initiated on amitriptyline 50 mg ON, 4 days ago.

Drug interactions

A   bradycardia
B   hyperkalaemia
C   hypertensive crisis
D   hypoglycaemia
E   hypokalaemia
F   hyponatraemia
G   increased risk of bleeding
H   ventricular arrhythmias

For questions 9–16

For the patients described below, select the single most likely possible consequence of the drug interaction. Each option may be used once, more than once or not at all.

9   A 43-year-old patient has been taking fluoxetine 40 mg capsules OD. He has newly been prescribed diclofenac 50 mg tablets TDS.

10   A 54-year-old patient has been taking escitalopam 20 mg tablets OD. She has newly been prescribed quinine tablets.

11   A 56-year-old patient has been taking salbutamol 100 mcg two puffs QDS PRN. She has newly been prescribed furosemide 20 mg tablets OM.

12   A 61-year-old patient has been taking amiodarone 200 mg tablets daily. He has newly been prescribed diltiazem MR 60 mg tablets BD.

13   A 61-year-old patient has been taking furosemide 40 mg tablets daily. He has newly been prescribed amisulpiride 200 mg BD.

14   A 46-year-old patient has been taking metformin 500 mg tablets TDS and gliclazide 80 mg tablets daily. She has newly been prescribed intravenous chloramphenicol to query meningitis.

15   A 46-year-old patient has been taking spironolactone 100 mg tablets OD. He has newly been prescribed ciclosporin 7.5 mg BD.

16   A 48-year-old patient has been taking propranolol 100 mg OD. She has newly been prescribed an adrenaline injection because she has been found to have a severe peanut allergy.

Analgesics

A   diamorphine powder for solution for injection
B   diclofenac suppositories
C   ibuprofen liquid
D   morphine sulfate tablets
E   oxycodone injection
F   paracetamol tablets
G   pethidine injection
H   tramadol capsules

For questions 17–23

For the scenarios described below, select the single most suitable analgesic from the list above. Each option may be used once, more than once or not at all.

17   A 37-year-old man, who has severe pain from bone metastases, receiving palliative care in a hospice, following advanced prostate cancer. He is unable to swallow and has previously not tolerated oxycodone. All his regular medications have been withdrawn.

18   A 23-year-old woman, who has no long-term medical conditions and no drug allergies, presents at the pharmacy with a pain in her elbow after a weekend of playing golf. On further questioning you feel it appropriate for her to be treated. She tells you that she is 26 weeks' pregnant.

19   A 52-year-old woman who has chronic back pain and has previously had spinal surgery to replace one of her vertebrae. She has previously had a gastric ulcer due to NSAID usage. She has tried morphine sulfate in the past, but does not like that 'feeling of detachment' associated with it, and does not want to try it again because she has also heard people become addicted to it and is worried about that happening to her. She is currently on the maximum dose of co-codamol 30/500 mg tablets.

20 A 72-year-old man who has severe pain from lung cancer. He is currently in a hospice and is able to take medication orally. All of his regular medication has been withdrawn. He has a previous history of cardiac disease and COPD.

21 A 32-year-old woman who has severe pain during childbirth. She is currently on the labour ward and has no known drug allergies. She takes levothyroxine 50 mcg OD.

22 A 9-year-old girl who has pain and fever associated with influenza. She has no known drug allergies and has recently been prescribed chloramphenicol eye drops to treat bacterial conjunctivitis. Her mother tells you that her daughter is unable to swallow tablets.

23 A 42-year-old man who is having surgery for a severe fractured leg. He has previously had a severe reaction to opioids. He is on no other medication and is otherwise fit and well. An alternative postoperative analgesic has been requested to be administered while the patient is sedated.

Cough and cold

A codeine linctus
B co-codamol 8/500 mg tablets
C guaifenesin
D ibuprofen liquid
E paracetamol liquid
F phenylephrine
G saline nose drops
H warm lemon and honey drinks

For questions 24–30

For the scenarios described below, select the single most suitable cough and cold medicine from the list above. Each option may be used once, more than once or not at all.

24 A 4-year-old girl who has a dry cough and blocked nose. She has had these symptoms for 2 days. She is on no other medication and is not allergic to anything. Her mother would like to know what is suitable to treat the dry cough.

25 A 3-year-old boy who has nasal congestion. He has had these symptoms for 3 days. He is on no other medication and is not allergic to anything. His father would like to know what is suitable to treat the nasal congestion.

26 A 17-year-old boy who has nasal congestion. He has had these symptoms for 3 days. He is on no other medication and is not allergic to anything. His mother would like to know what is suitable to treat the nasal congestion.

27 A 16-year-old boy who has a dry cough. He has had these symptoms for 5 days. He is on no other medication and is not allergic to anything. His mother would like to know what is suitable to treat the dry cough.

28 A 6-year-old girl who has a fever associated with a cold. She has had these symptoms for 3 days. She is on insulin therapy and takes salbutamol 100 mcg, two puffs QDS PRN. She is not allergic to anything. Her mother would like to know what is suitable to treat the fever.

29 A 3-year-old girl who has fever associated with chickenpox. She has had these symptoms for 2 days. She not allergic to anything and has no past medical history. Her mother would like to know what is suitable to treat the fever.

30 A 2-year-old boy who has fever associated with a common cold. He has had these symptoms for 3 days. He is not allergic to anything. He has moderate renal impairment. His mother would like to know what is suitable to treat the fever.

SECTION D

Oksana Pyzik

In this section, for each numbered question, select the one lettered option that most closely corresponds to the answer. Within each group of questions each lettered option may be used once, more than once or not at all.

Endocrinology – diabetes

A   acarbose
B   canagliflozin
C   liraglutide
D   metformin
E   nateglinide
F   pioglitazone
G   tolbutamide
H   vildagliptin

For questions 1–3

For the patients described below, select the single most likely anti-diabetic drug from the list above. Each option may be used once, more than once or not at all.

1   A 62-year-old woman with type 2 diabetes, asthma, arthritis and deep vein thrombosis, who has insufficient glycaemic control. She leads a sedentary lifestyle and, according to the SCR, she weighs 94 kg and is 160 cm tall. The patient notes reveal that she has already been prescribed first-line and second-line anti-diabetic therapies but has struggled to lose weight and reach target HbA1c levels. The GP has issued a new prescription for a human glucagon-like peptide-1 (GLP-1) analogue produced by recombinant DNA technology in *Saccharomyces cerevisiae*. You counsel her to inject the medicine once daily at any time of day (before or after meals) and to rotate injection sites. The prescriber has advised that, if she has not lost at least 5% of her initial body weight after 12 weeks on the 3.0 mg/day dose, the treatment will be discontinued.

2   A 58-year-old man with poorly controlled type 2 diabetes has been prescribed a meglitinide drug as an adjunct to stimulate insulin secretion. The patient was previously taking the maximum tolerated

dose of an anti-diabetic drug as a monotherapy, but failed to achieve adequate glycaemic control despite making significant lifestyle changes. The newly prescribed drug has a rapid onset of action and short duration of activity. This drug can be used flexibly around mealtimes and adjusted to fit around individual eating habits, which is beneficial to this patient's lifestyle.

3   A 55-year-old female with type 2 diabetes taking a sodium-glucose co-transporter 2 (SGLT2) inhibitor developed the following symptoms: rapid weight loss, nausea and vomiting, abdominal pain, fast and deep breathing, sleepiness, a sweet smell to the breath, a sweet or metallic taste in the mouth, and a different odour to urine and sweat. Tests reveal raised ketone levels confirming diabetic ketoacidosis, and treatment is immediately discontinued.

Anaesthetics

    A   desflurane
    B   etomidate
    C   ketamine
    D   neostigmine
    E   nitrous oxide
    F   propofol
    G   sevoflurane
    H   thiopental sodium

For questions 4–10

For the drugs described below, match the single most likely anaesthetic from the list above. Each option may be used once, more than once or not at all.

4   This is an anaesthetic agent used for diagnostic and surgical procedures, although now rarely used. It is sometimes used as a paediatric anaesthetic for treating serial burns dressings, which requires repeated administration. Recovery is relatively slow and there is a high incidence of extraneous muscle movements. The main disadvantage is the high incidence of hallucinations, nightmares and other transient psychotic effects.

5   This is the most widely used intravenous anaesthetic and can be used for induction or maintenance of anaesthesia in adults and children. It is also associated with rapid recovery and has less of a hangover effect than other intravenous anaesthetics.

6   This is unsatisfactory as a sole anaesthetic owing to a lack of potency, but it is useful as part of a combination of drugs because it allows a significant reduction in dosage. Hypoxia can occur immediately following administration. It should not be given continuously for longer than 24 hours or more frequently than every 4 days without close supervision and haematological monitoring.

7   This is an intravenous agent associated with rapid recovery without a hangover effect. It causes less hypotension than other intravenous anaesthetics. It suppresses adrenocortical function, particularly during continuous administration, and it should not be used for maintenance of anaesthesia. It should be used with caution in patients with underlying adrenal insufficiency, e.g. those with sepsis.

8   This is a barbiturate that is used for induction of anaesthesia, but it has no analgesic properties. Induction is generally smooth and rapid, but dose-related cardiovascular and respiratory depression can occur. Awakening from a moderate dose of this drug is rapid because the drug redistributes into other tissues, particularly fat. However, metabolism is slow and the sedative effects can persist for 24 hours. Repeated doses have a cumulative effect and recovery is much slower.

9   This is a rapidly acting volatile liquid anaesthetic that is used extensively. It is non-irritant and therefore often used for inhalational induction of anaesthesia; it has little effect on heart rhythm compared with other volatile liquid anaesthetics. However, it can interact with carbon dioxide absorbents to form compound A, a potentially nephrotoxic vinyl ether.

10 This is administered after surgery and used specifically for reversal of non-depolarising competitive blockade. It acts within 1 minute of intravenous injection and its effects last for 20–30 minutes.

Antimalarials

A   choloroquine
B   doxycycline
C   *Lariam* (mefloquine)

D   *Malarone* (proguanil with atovaquone)
E   primaquine
F   pyrimethamine
G   *Riamet* (artemether with lumefantrine)
H   quinine

> For questions 11–15
>
> For the drugs described below, match the single most likely antimalarial from the list above. Each option may be used once, more than once or not at all.

11 It is no longer recommended for the treatment of falciparum malaria due to extensive resistance. It is also not recommended if the infective species is unknown or if the infection is mixed.

12 In addition to taking precautions with mosquito nets and use of insect repellents, advise the patient to wear sunscreen due to drug-induced photosensitivity.

13 Avoid in patients with a history of epilepsy, depression or other mental health disorders.

14 If used for malaria prophylaxis, this antimalarial should be administered 24–48 hours prior to entering a malaria-endemic area, continued during the period of the stay, and then taken for another 7 days after leaving the area. It is effective against drug-sensitive and drug-resistant *P. falciparum* and it is especially recommended for prophylaxis and treatment of *P. falciparum* malaria where the pathogen may be resistant to other antimalarials.

15 When used for malaria prophylaxis this antimalarial should be given once weekly, always on the same day. It is recommended to start chemoprophylaxis 10 days before departure to ensure administration is well tolerated. Subsequent doses should be taken once a week (on a fixed day). Treatment should then be continued for 4 weeks after leaving a malaria-endemic area (the minimum treatment period is 6 weeks). The maximum recommended duration of administration is 12 months.

Antiepileptics

A   carbamazepine
B   lamotrigine
C   lorazepam
D   phenytoin sodium
E   primidone
F   sodium valproate
G   topirimate
H   zonisamide

For questions 16–23

For the patients/statements described below, match the single most likely antiepileptic from the list above. Each option may be used once, more than once or not at all.

16 This undergoes biotransformation into two metabolites, phenobarbitone and phenylethylmalonamide, which have anticonvulsant activity.

17 A 45-year-old man has started treatment with an anti-epileptic and has developed acute myopia with secondary angle-closure glaucoma within 1 month of starting treatment.

18 A 53-year-old man develops kidney stones while taking this anti-epileptic medicine.

19 A 37-year-old woman with epilepsy has had her drug regimen changed with an optimum response at a plasma concentration of 4–12 mg/L (17–50 micromol/L).

20 A 34-year-old woman has a seizure that lasts 6 minutes and receives treatment intravenously. The patient should be monitored for respiratory depression and hypotension.

21 Patients taking this drug or their carers should be told how to recognise signs and symptoms of pancreatitis, and advised to seek immediate medical attention if symptoms such as abdominal pain, nausea or vomiting develop.

22 An 18-year-old young man has been newly diagnosed with epilepsy
    and has commenced treatment with this anti-epileptic. You counsel
    the patient to recognise the signs of hepatotoxicity as liver dysfunction
    is associated with this drug and is most likely to occur within the
    first 6 months of treatment. Raised liver enzymes during treatment are
    usually transient, but the patient should be monitored for liver function
    and prothrombin time until levels return to normal.

23 This anti-epileptic is highly teratogenic. Infants exposed to this drug
    in utero are at a high risk of serious developmental disorders (up to
    30–40%) and congenital malformations (approximately 11% risk). It
    should not be used in female children, females of childbearing potential
    or during pregnancy unless alternative treatments are ineffective or not
    tolerated. Female patients and their carers must be counselled on the
    risks of treatment during pregnancy.

Vaccines

    A   cholera vaccine
    B   diphtheria vaccine
    C   hepatitis A vaccine
    D   hepatitis B vaccine
    E   human papillomavirus vaccine
    F   rabies vaccine
    G   rotavirus vaccine
    H   yellow fever vaccine

For questions 24–27

For the scenarios/statements described below, match the single most
likely vaccine from the list above. Each option may be used once, more
than once or not at all.

24 A 6-year-old boy is prescribed an oral vaccine. You counsel the carer
    to dissolve effervescent sodium bicarbonate granules in a glassful of
    water or chlorinated water (approximately 150 mL). Discard half,
    approximately 75 mL, of the solution, then add vaccine suspension to
    make one dose and drink within 2 hours. Food, drink and other oral
    medicines should be avoided for 1 hour before and after vaccination.

25 This vaccine may be administered from the age of 9 years for the
    prevention of premalignant genital lesions (cervical, vulvar and vaginal),
    premalignant anal lesions, cervical cancers, anal cancers and genital
    warts (condyloma acuminata).

26 A 6-week-old infant is prescribed a live oral vaccine against gastroenteritis. The second dose is administered 4 weeks later.

27 A zoologist requires this immunisation as a booster dose due to his work with primates.

Laboratory tests

A alanine aminotransferase (ALT)
B alkaline phosphatase (ALP)
C aspartate aminotransferase (AST)
D bilirubin
E C-reactive protein
F creatinine
G HbA1c
H Urea

For questions 28–32

For the scenarios/statements described below, match the single most likely laboratory test from the list above. Each option may be used once, more than once or not at all.

28 A 68-year-old man who may be suffering from cardiovascular disease.

29 A 51-year-old man who may have Crigler–Najjar syndrome.

30 Test results are a value that corresponds to a 3-month average.

31 Normal range is between 60 and 125 micromol/L.

32 Normal range is between 3 and 7 mmol/L.

Obstetrics and gynaecology

A *Cerazette* (desogestrel 75 mcg)
B *Copper T 380A*
C *Evra* (ethinylestradiol 33.9 mcg/24 h and norelgestromin 203 mcg/24 h)
D *Loestrin* (ethinylestradiol 20 mcg/norethisterone acetate 1 mg)
E *Microgynon 30* ED (ethinylestradiol 30 mcg/levonorgestrel 150 mcg)

F   *Mifegyne* (mifepristone)
G   *Syntocinon* (oxytocin)
H   *EllaOne* (ulipristal acetate)

> For questions 33–40
>
> For the scenarios/statements described below, match the single most likely drug from the list above. Each option may be used once, more than once or not at all.

33 A 19-year-old young woman brings in a prescription for a combined oral contraceptive pill that is a monophasic low-strength 21-day preparation.

34 A 25-year-old young woman collects a prescription for a combined oral contraceptive pill that is a monophasic standard strength 28-day preparation.

35 A 21-year-old woman asks about how to use the contraceptive patch. You advise her to apply the patch once weekly for 3 weeks, followed by a 7-day patch-free interval. Subsequent courses repeated after a 7-day patch-free interval during which withdrawal bleeding occurs.

36 This is prescribed for women who cannot tolerate oestrogen-containing contraceptives.

37 A 35-year-old woman is undergoing an abortion. She is prescribed an anti-progestogenic steroid that sensitises the myometrium to prostaglandin-induced contractions and ripens the cervix. A single dose is taken for termination of pregnancy, followed by administration of a prostaglandin.

38 Take 30 mg as a single dose as soon as possible after coitus, but no later than after 120 hours.

39 This is administered by slow intravenous infusion, using an infusion pump, to induce or augment labour, usually in conjunction with amniotomy. Uterine activity must be monitored carefully and hyperstimulation avoided. Large doses may result in excessive fluid retention.

40 May be used to control bleeding due to incomplete miscarriage or abortion and is administered intramuscularly. The dose is adjusted according to the patient's condition and blood loss.

Calculation questions

Ryan Hamilton

1   One of the nurses calls you from the neonatal unit regarding parenteral nutrition for one of her patients. The nurse needs to make up a 50 mL syringe containing 27.5% glucose for IV infusion. Earlier in the day your pharmacy department supplied the ward with a 50 mL vial of glucose 50% and a 100 mL bag of glucose 20%, both of which will need to be used to make the required infusion.
    What volume (mL) of glucose 50% will the nurse need to use? Give your answer to one decimal place.

2   You are working on the respiratory ward and the medical team want to prescribe piperacillin/tazobactam for one of their bronchiectasis patients, Mrs U, an 81-year-old woman weighing 47 kg. Her serum creatinine is 138 micromol/L and her eGFR has been reported as 31 ml/min per 1.73 m^2 through the laboratory results system.
    You decide to calculate Mrs U's renal function (mL/min) using the Cockcroft and Gault formula. Give your answer to one decimal place.

$$CrCl = \frac{(140 - age\,[years]) \times Weight\,(kg) \times F}{SeCr}$$

    where F is 1.23 for males and 1.04 for females.

3   Miss C comes into your pharmacy with a prescription for her 9-year-old daughter, who has been prescribed flucloxacillin 125 mg/5 mL suspension at a dose of 250 mg QDS for 7 days.
    Given that, when the suspension is made up it has an expiry date of 7 days, how many 100 mL bottles should you supply?

4   Mr G has been admitted to your ward with delirium and has been refusing his medicines. Before admission he was taking digoxin 250 mcg every morning and the medical team feel it necessary to administer this parenterally as he now has tachycardia. You note the fact that oral digoxin is only 63% bioavailable and an IV dose of 250 mcg may be inappropriate.
Given that intravenous digoxin is available as 500 mcg/2 mL ampoules, calculate the equivalent daily dose (mcg) of IV digoxin to one decimal place.

5   Mrs K is suffering from heart failure. On medical review she has responded well to the intravenous loading dose of digoxin and the medical team want to place her on long-term oral therapy, aiming for a serum digoxin of 2.0 mcg/L (acceptable range of 1.5–2.0 mcg/L). You obtain the following information from her notes:

Weight: 95 kg	**Height:** 5'5''	**Age:** 71 years
HR: 73 BPM	**BP:** 133/81	**Temp:** 36.4°C
Creatinine: 93 micromol/L	**K⁺:** 3.6 mmol/L	**Urea:** 4.1 mmol/L

Calculate the daily oral dose (mcg) that Mrs K should initially be prescribed, accounting for the fact that digoxin tablets come in 62.5 mcg, 125 mcg and 250 mcg strengths, and are approximately 63% bioavailable.

$$C_{pss} = \frac{(BA \times D)}{(DigCl \times t)}$$

Non-heart failure DigCl (L/h) = $(0.06 \times CrCl \,[mL/min])$
$+ (0.05 \times IBW \,[kg])$

Heart failure DigCl (L/h) = $(0.053 \times CrCl \,[mL/min])$
$+ (0.02 \times IBW \,[kg])$

Male IBW = 50 kg + 2.3 kg
for every inch over 5 ft

Female IBW = 45.5 kg + 2.3 kg
for every inch over 5 ft

$$CrCl = \frac{(140 - age\,[yrs]) \times IBW\,[kg] \times F}{SeCr}$$

where IBW is ideal body weight, BA is the bioavailability, and F is 1.23 for males, and 1.04 for females.

6 You have received a prescription for Mr W, a 96-year-old man, who is receiving end-of-life care, is developing swallowing problems and has poor vascular access. His consultant has written a prescription for twenty-eight (28) 1 g suppositories, each containing morphine sulfate 12.5 mg, for breakthrough pain, which you need to make up extemporaneously. You find the displacement value of morphine sulfate is 1.6 and you decide to work out a formula to make an excess of two suppositories.

Calculate how much (g) *Witepsol* (to be used as the base) you would need. Give your answer to two decimal places.

7 Mrs H is due to commence a course of chemotherapy and the consultants would like to dose her by body surface area. You look at Mrs H's notes and find that she is 1.23 m tall and weighs 63 kg.

$$BSA\ (m^2) = ([\text{height (cm)} \times \text{weight (kg)}] \div 3600)^{0.5}$$

Calculate Mrs H's body surface area (BSA, m^2) to one decimal place.

8 What weight (mg) of zinc oxide powder must you add to 30 g of 1% (w/w) zinc oxide cream to produce a cream of 5% (w/w)? Give your answer to one decimal place.

9 Mr E brings in a prescription for *Zomorph* (morphine sulfate modified-release) 60 mg capsules, with a prescribed regimen of 120 mg BD. He has also been prescribed *Oramorph* 10 mg/5 mL oral solution, 5 mg to be taken when needed for pain relief. You believe this dose to be too small and discuss breakthrough pain doses with the GP, who asks you what the maximum breakthrough dose of *Oramorph* would be for this patient.

Calculate the maximum breakthrough dose (mg) of *Oramorph* to the nearest whole milligram.

10 Miss L comes into your pharmacy with a new prescription from her dermatologist who has prescribed:

Dimethyl fumarate 120 mg PO MDU as per standard initiation regimen. Supply 8/52.

How many dimethyl fumarate 120 mg tablets will you need to supply to cover the prescribed course?
You can use the SPC for dimethyl fumarate to support your calculations: http://www.medicines.org.uk/emc/medicine/28593

11 Baby V is a patient on your paediatric ward suffering from hypocalcaemia and weighs 3.78 kg. On the ward round the consultant paediatrician would like to infuse Baby V with 0.5 mmol/kg of calcium over 24 hours and asks you to support the nurses to make up an appropriate IV infusion.

You find the following molecular masses for compounds commonly used to make up intravenous infusions including parenteral nutrition.

Formula	g/mol
$CaCl_2$	110.88
$CaCl_2 \cdot 2H_2O$	147.01
KCl	74.55
$MgCl_2$	95.21
NaCl	58.44

How many millilitres of calcium chloride dihydrate solution 13.4% (w/v) should be used in this infusion? Give your answer to the nearest 0.1 mL.

12 Mrs U has been diagnosed with an acute flare of ulcerative colitis and has been prescribed prednisolone. You are given her prescription and note she has been placed on a weaning dose of prednisolone. She is required to take a high dose of prednisolone 60 mg OD for 14 days then wean by 5 mg every week until zero.

How many 5 mg prednisolone tablets should you supply to ensure that Mrs U can complete her course?

13 Mr G has been admitted to your endocrine ward with an infected diabetic foot ulcer and suspected osteomyelitis. The endocrine registrar has prescribed an IV infusion of vancomycin 2000 mg every 12 hours, which the nurses will make up to 500 mL using 0.9% sodium chloride or 5% glucose.

What is the fastest rate (mL/h) at which the infusion device can be set? Give your answer to one decimal place.

You may use the SPC for vancomycin to help you answer this question: www.medicines.org.uk/emc/medicine/21291

14 Mr Z has been newly diagnosed with pulmonary multi-drug-resistant (MDR) TB and his medical team are going to add in prothionamide 15 mg/kg once daily to his treatment regimen. On the ward round

you note that Mr Z weighs only 49 kg and has an eGFR >90 mL/min. You consult the TB drug monograph website (www.tbdrugmonographs .co.uk) and find the following information for prothionamide:

PROTHIONAMIDE

Please note prothionamide is not licensed in the UK.

Prothionamide is a thioamide, and is considered to be interchangeable with ethionamide (currently not available in the UK).

DOSAGE

Adult & paediatric doses are the same per kg.

Adults: 15–20 mg/kg (max. 1 g) once daily (oral).

Once-daily dosing is preferred to maximise peak levels, particularly for daily doses ≤750 mg. Consider twice-daily dosing if patients are unable to tolerate once-daily regimens.

Children: 15–20 mg/kg (max. 1 g) once daily (oral).

Once-daily dosing is preferred to maximise peak levels, particularly for daily doses ≤750 mg. Consider twice-daily dosing if patients are unable to tolerate once-daily regimens.

WHO advise a once-daily dosing regimen if tolerated (to maximise peak levels), but twice-daily regimens may be required if unable to tolerate.

Prothionamide should be taken with or after meals to reduce gastrointestinal adverse effects. Most patients also require gradual dose escalation, i.e. for adults: initially 250 mg once a day, increasing by 250 mg every 3 to 5 days.

All patients must be prescribed pyridoxine whilst receiving prothionamide. The usual adult dose ranges from 50 mg to 100 mg daily, up to 50 mg per 250 mg of prothionamide.

PREPARATIONS

Oral: 250-mg tablets (unlicensed medicine).

Source: http://www.tbdrugmonographs.co.uk/prothionamide.html [accessed 12/2/2017]

Knowing that the tablets can be split in half, what total daily dose (mg) should the medical team prescribe for Mr Z?

15 Mr A comes to see you about losing weight and would like to try orlistat. During the consultation you take his weight and measurements and find that Mr A is 156 cm tall and weighs 103.5 kg.
How much weight (kg) does Mr A need to lose in order to reach a healthy BMI of 24 kg/m²? Give your answer to one decimal place.

16 Mrs P has been admitted to your ward and has had a nasogastric tube fitted. While undertaking her medication history you note she was taking phenytoin capsules 200 mg twice daily to control her epilepsy. The medical team have prescribed phenytoin oral suspension, which you know is not bioequivalent. You find that 100 mg of phenytoin sodium (present in the capsules) is equivalent to 92 mg of the phenytoin base (present in the oral suspension).
How many millilitres of phenytoin 30 mg/5 mL oral suspension should Mrs P take for each dose? Give your answer to the nearest whole millilitre.

17 Mr W is a man who has been coming to your community pharmacy for 10 years to collect prescriptions for carbamazepine 300 mg BD (as 100 mg and 200 mg immediate-release tablets) for his epilepsy. He has recently suffered a stroke and the hospital has changed him to carbamazepine rectally until his swallowing improves.
What dose (mg) of carbamazepine suppositories would you expect Mr W to be using for each dose? Give your answer to the nearest whole milligram.
You can use the carbamazepine monograph in the BNF to help you answer this question.

18 You receive a prescription for Miss L who is being newly started on gabapentin for neuropathic pain. The prescription is for the standard induction regimen of 300 mg OD on day 1, then 300 mg BD on day 2 and 300 mg TDS thereafter.
How many gabapentin 300 mg capsules do you need to dispense if the total duration on the prescription is 14 days?

19 You are a quality control (QC) pharmacist working in the QC labs for your hospital's manufacturing unit. You are testing the concentration of clonidine in a batch of solution to determine whether it fits within the limits allowed for a desired concentration of 50 mcg/5 mL.
Your QC department has produced the following calibration curve for clonidine oral solution utilising UV-visible spectrophotometry at 271 nm.

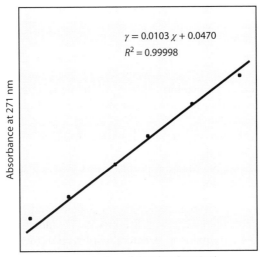

$\gamma = 0.0103\,\chi + 0.0470$

$R^2 = 0.99998$

Concentration of clonidine (mcg/mL)

If UV-visible absorbance at 271 nm for this batch is 0.151, what is the concentration (mcg/5 mL) of clonidine in the solution? Give your answer to two decimal places.

20 Mr M has been diagnosed with infective endocarditis and the micro-biologist has advised commencing benzylpenicillin until cultures and sensitivities are available. The recommended regimen is 2.4 g IV every 4 hours, given in 100 mL of 5% glucose infused over 60 minutes. His medical team are concerned about the sodium content of this product and ask you to calculate how much sodium the patient will receive.

How many millimoles of sodium will Mr M receive every 24 hours on this regimen? Give your answer to two decimal places.

You may use the SPC for benzylpenicillin to help you with your calculations: www.medicines.org.uk/emc/medicine/32345

21 Mr J is taking morphine sulfate *MST continus* 30 mg and 60 mg tablets at a total dose of 90 mg BD. While his pain is fairly well controlled, his oncology team are concerned that he will struggle to take these tablets in the near future, and decide to change him to a fentanyl transdermal patch.

What strength (mcg/h patch) of fentanyl 72-hour transdermal patch should be prescribed for Mr J?

You can use the Prescribing in palliative care section of the BNF to support your working.

22 Miss Q is going travelling and her GP calls you to discuss malaria prophylaxis as she will be visiting Asia. Miss Q will start her journey in the city of Vientiane in Laos where she will stay for 3 days. She will then travel west through the forests to undertake 4 weeks' of conservation work, before arriving in Chiang Mai in Thailand, where she will stay for 10 days. You confirm that it will be unlikely for Miss L to avoid exposure to the sun, so you suggest that the GP prescribes *Malarone* tablets once daily.

What is the maximum number of *Malarone* tablets needed to protect Miss Q during this trip?

You may use the Malaria, prophylaxis section of the BNF to help you with this question.

23 Mr K is one of your cystic fibrosis patients and is being discharged on IV ceftazidime 2 g every 8 hours, to be administered through the local OPAT (outpatient parenteral antibacterial therapy) scheme. Each ceftazidime 2 g vial is reconstituted with 10 mL sodium chloride 0.9% and given as a bolus. The nurses will also flush the patient's line with 3–5 mL sodium chloride 0.9% before and after each dose is given.

How many ampoules of 10 mL sodium chloride 0.9% should be supplied to sufficiently cover a 4-week course? Give your answer to the nearest five ampoules.

24 Mr D has been admitted to your endocrine unit with diabetic ketoacidosis requiring urgent treatment. He has been prescribed a 500 mL infusion of sodium bicarbonate 1.26% to be given over 6 hours. You inform the medical team to monitor his sodium levels closely due to him having severe renal impairment.

How much sodium (mmol) will Mr D be receiving from this treatment? Give your answer as a whole number.

You may use the BNF monograph for sodium bicarbonate to support your working.

25 Mr R calls you up to ask for some advice. His 4-month-old son, Sam, has recently been prescribed long-term oral hydrocortisone 4 mg at 8am then 1 mg at 12pm and 4pm. He has been supplied with 10 mg hydrocortisone tablets, which he was advised to crush and disperse, but he is not sure how much to administer. Hydrocortisone tablets are scored so you advise him to disperse half a tablet in 10 mL of water.

How much of this dispersion should be given for the morning dose? Give your answer to the nearest whole millilitre.

26 Mrs N has been prescribed oral capecitabine at a dose of 1.25 g/m^2 twice daily for the next 14 days. The prescription states that her height is 1.53 m and her weight 61.87 kg.

Given that capecitabine tablets are available in 150 mg, 300 mg and 500 mg strengths, what dose of capecitabine (mg) should Mrs N be supplied with for each dose?

BSA (m^2) = ([height (cm) × weight (kg)] ÷ 3600)$^{0.5}$

27 Mrs C is required to take co-trimoxazole for prophylaxis against *Pneumocystis jirovecii* (*Pneumocystis carinii*) infections at a dose of 960 mg each morning and evening on Mondays, Wednesdays and Fridays. Your pharmacy only stocks the 480 mg strength of co-trimoxazole. How many 480 mg co-trimoxazole tablets are required to cover a 12-week period?

28 Miss E is a 32-year-old woman, weighing 63 kg, who has been admitted to your emergency department with confusion after ingesting approximately 110 tablets of co-codamol 8/500. The medical team take a sample of blood to test for plasma-paracetamol concentrations, but decide to initiate an acetylcysteine infusion before the plasma concentration results are back.
How much acetylcysteine (g) will Miss E receive if she is given all three infusions of acetylcysteine? Give your answer to one decimal place.
You may use the Emergency treatment of poisoning – paracetamol section of the BNF to support your calculations.

29 Mr O is taking warfarin for antiphospholipid syndrome and has just been to the anticoagulation clinic to get his INR checked. He presents you with his yellow book, which advises Mr O to take 3 mg every day except Sunday and Wednesday when he will take 2 mg.
How many packs of 28 warfarin 1 mg tablets do you need to supply for 4 weeks?

30 You are working within the antimicrobial pharmacist team in your hospital and are looking to make cost savings across commonly used drugs. You decide to determine what cost savings can be achieved by switching from meropenem 1 g TDS for 5 days to meropenem 500 mg QDS for 5 days.
Your purchasing department obtains packs of 10 meropenem 500 mg vials at a cost of £76.90 and packs of 10 meropenem 1 g vials at a cost of £153.50.
Calculate the expected cost saving per 100 patients by undertaking this switch. Give your answer to the nearest whole pound sterling (£).

SECTION B

Simon Harris

1   A 52-year-old woman presents a prescription for prednisolone tablets 5 mg. She has been prescribed a reducing dose after taking prednisolone for the last 8 weeks to suppress an allergic disorder. Her initial dose of 60 mg daily is to be taken for another 10 days. At the end of the 10 days she is to reduce her daily dose by 5 mg once each week until the course is finished. You have in stock 147 tablets, and agree to supply her with 112 tablets to allow you to keep some for any further patients this afternoon. You will then owe her the rest, which you should have in stock tomorrow. How many tablets will you owe the patient when she returns tomorrow?

2   A palliative care patient has been set up with a diamorphine infusion in their home, which delivers the drug over 24 hours. She is currently receiving a dose of 320 mg over a 24-hour period, using a syringe pump that is calibrated to 36 mm/24 h. She is now complaining of breakthrough pain and, after calculating the amount of additional analgesia required along with the palliative care team, you agree to increase the rate of infusion to 48 mm/24 h. How much diamorphine (mg) will the patient now receive at this increased rate over 24 hours? Give your answer to the nearest 5 mg.

3   You have been asked to prepare 25 suppositories for a young child. The paediatrician would like each suppository to be prepared in a 2 g mould, with each containing 125 mg paracetamol. The displacement value of paracetamol is 1.5, and the base to be used is glycerol. You know from experience that it's always worth making extra, and so decide to increase the batch size by 20%. What weight of glycerol (g) will be required to prepare all the suppositories, including the additional 20%? Give your answer to one decimal place.

4   A 7-month-old baby with a wheeze and a chesty cough has been examined by a specialist pharmacist at a paediatric clinic. The baby is diagnosed with a severe bacterial chest infection and prescribed co-amoxiclav 125/31 oral suspension. The baby weighs 7 kg and has been given a dose of 0.5 mL/kg three times a day for 14 days.
    What volume (mL) of co-amoxiclav oral suspension 125 mg/31mg per 5 mL should be dispensed to supply enough for the first 7 days of treatment? Give your answer to the nearest 5 mL.

5 Mrs P has chronic renal failure and is today attending the hospital for her haemodialysis appointment. She is found to have anaemia, and the doctor prescribes a course of subcutaneous epoetin zeta. Epoetin zeta is to be given at a dose of 60 units/kg three times a week for the first 4 weeks, 80 units/kg three times a week for the following 4 weeks and then 100 units/kg three times a week as a maintenance dose. Mrs P weighs 75 kg. What is the total amount of epoetin zeta (units) that Mrs P will receive for her first 12 weeks of treatment?

6 You are working as a practice pharmacist for your local CCG, and have been asked to review patients on unlicensed cholecalciferol (vitamin D). You have been advised to change these patients, if appropriate, to the licensed versions of the medicine instead. You run a search on your computer, which produces the following results:

Drug	No. of patients	Cost per patient per month
Cholecalciferol 800 units, tablets	25	£29.60
Cholecalciferol 3200 units, tablets	13	£58.90
Cholecalciferol 25 000 units, liquid	5	£112.50

The licensed versions of these medicines are listed below, which are given to patients at the same dose as those listed in the table above:

Item	Cost per patient per month
Cholecalciferol 800 units, tablets	£3.60
Cholecalciferol 3200 units, tablets	£13.32
Cholecalciferol 25 000 units, liquid	£4.45

Calculate the total savings that could be made per month, to the nearest pound, if all these patients are successfully reviewed and placed on to the licensed medications.

7 Mr N is being treated for alcohol withdrawal at a private clinic, and has been prescribed a reducing dose of chlordiazepoxide. Mr N's consultant would like him to take his daily dose in four divided doses, starting

with 200 mg daily for the first 2 days, and then gradually reducing the dose of chlordiazepoxide by 25 mg a day until he has stopped. It has been decided to issue Mr N with 5 mg tablets, which he is happy to take. After looking at your supplier's website, you find the price is £19.50 for 50 tablets. How much will the private prescription for Mr N be, assuming you follow your private prescription pricing guidelines, which are to first add a 30% mark-up and then a £4.50 dispensing fee? Give your answer to the nearest pound.

8   Cefalexin powder for reconstitution into an injection has a displacement volume of 0.8 mL/g. To reconstitute the injection, 12 mL of water is added to 500 mg of the powder. What is the final concentration (% w/v) of the reconstituted solution?

9   Within the dispensary at the hospital where you work, there is a stock solution of povidone–iodine with a concentration of 48% (w/v). Before being sent for use in the theatre for skin disinfection, it must be diluted to an appropriate concentration to avoid the risk of theatre staff applying it as the concentrate.
The surgery team apply the povidone–iodine to the patients at a concentration of 12.5% (w/v). Due to stability issues, you supply them with an intermediate strength, such that the surgery team have to dilute this intermediate solution 1 in 2 to get the correct concentration immediately before use. What is the concentration (% w/v) of the intermediate solution that you supply to the surgery team?

10   You are asked to prepare 4325 mL of a magnesium sulfate solution such that, when diluted 15 times, a 1 in 6000 solution is obtained. What weight of magnesium sulfate, in kilograms, will you need? Give your answer to two decimal places.

11   An injection solution of botulinum toxin type B contains 2500 units/ 0.5 mL of active ingredient. A hospital manufacturing unit is creating batches of 2 mL injection solution in ampoules to supply to local hospitals. Each batch size is 20 ampoules plus an extra 15% for quality control (QC) batch testing. How many units of botulinum toxin are needed to prepare two batches' worth?

12   You have been asked to supply tramadol suppositories using theobroma oil as a base for a 15-year-old girl who has had an operation to remove her appendix. The suppositories will be made using a 3.5 g mould and each suppository will contain 100 mg tramadol. You need to supply

30 suppositories, plus 20% extra for quality assurance (QA) checks. Given that the displacement value of tramadol in theobroma oil is 0.8, how much base (g) will be required to prepare the full quantity, including the additional for QA checks? Give your answer to one decimal place.

13 You have been asked to prepare 450 mL of an oral formulation for a patient on your ward. You have in stock all the items required, except the codeine phosphate 30 mg tablets, which you would normally crush to a fine powder, and then add to the mixture. In the dispensary you only have codeine phosphate 15 mg tablets available, which you decide will be appropriate to use considering the patient requires the medicine urgently. The formulation is to be prepared according to the following formula:

> Codeine phosphate: one 30 mg tablet
> Zinc oxide 50 mg
> Ascorbic acid 10 mg
> Orange syrup 3.5 mL
> Water up to 12.5 mL

What quantity of codeine phosphate 15 mg tablets will you need to make the required formulation?

14 Whilst working as a pharmacist in a GP practice, you've been asked to review patients with asthma who may be suitable for a dose reduction. You highlight 12 patients on *Seretide 250 Evohaler* who may be stepped down to *Seretide 125 Evohaler*, and 7 patients who are on *Symbicort 400/12 Turbohaler* who may be stepped down to *Symbicort 200/6 Turbohaler*.

Inhaler	Cost
Seretide 250 Evohaler (120 doses)	£59.48
Seretide 125 Evohaler (120 doses)	£35.00
Symbicort 400/12 Turbohaler (60 doses)	£38.00
Symbicort 200/6 Turbohaler (120 doses)	£38.00

Considering there are 4 months left within the financial year, the surgery business manager asks you what the forecasted savings would be if all the patients were successfully stepped down.

Counting 30 days as 1 month, what is the total saving (£) for the practice over the next 4 months rounded to the nearest whole pound?

Assume all patients taking *Seretide* are using TWO puffs twice a day and all the patients taking *Symbicort* are using ONE inhalation twice a day.

15 You receive a prescription from a regular patient for *Nasonex* 50 mcg/dose 140 dose nasal spray. The directions on the prescription are as follows:

Rx. *Nasonex* nasal spray (mometasone furoate)

100 mcg OD for 3 days, then 50 mcg daily.

Apply to both nostrils

Mitte: 1 pack

How many days will the nasal spray last for this patient if they continue using it until it runs out?

16 A child is to receive erythromycin by intravenous infusion for a legionella infection. A vial containing 1 g erythromycin ethyl succinate powder for injection is to be reconstituted to produce 1.75 mL of injection. The displacement volume of erythromycin ethyl succinate is 0.05 mL/250 mg. How much water (mL) should be added to the powder to reconstitute the vial? Give your answer to one decimal place.

17 Chlorambucil has a half-life of 840 minutes. Immediately after administration to a patient, the plasma level is 126 mcg/mL. What would the plasma concentration (mcg/mL) be after 5 days and 20 hours? Give your answer to two decimal places.

18 A 26-year-old man who weighs 81 kg presents to hospital after ingesting ethylene glycol (anti-freeze) 2 hours ago. In accordance with hospital guidance, the consultant requests to use oral ethanol for the management of the overdose. The oral loading dose of ethanol (in the form of whisky, gin or vodka at 40% ethanol by volume) is 3.5 mL/kg. The pharmacy department supply gin at 25.5% ethanol by volume. How many millilitres of 25.5% gin will be required to provide a loading dose of ethanol for this patient? Give your answer to the nearest whole number.

19 A patient is prescribed *Nerisone* ointment to be applied twice a day for 2 weeks, to treat an exacerbation of their eczema. The cream is to be applied to their hands, scalp, face and neck.
A 30 g tube of *Nerisone* ointment contains 0.1% diflucortolone valerate. Two fingertip units (FTUs) is equivalent to approximately 1 g of topical steroid. To cover the hands, scalp, face and neck areas, the dermatologist has recommended that 7 FTUs are used per dose for this particular patient. What is the exact quantity (mg) of diflucortolone valerate that will have been applied to the affected areas in the first 14 days?

20 You have been asked to prepare 5 L of a potassium permanganate solution, such that the patient will dilute this 1 in 25 to obtain a 0.005% solution suitable for wound washing.
How many *Permitabs* 400-mg tablets will you dissolve in water before making the solution up to a final volume of 5 L with water? Give your answer to the nearest whole tablet.

21 A patient on your ward requires an intravenous infusion of nora-drenaline for acute hypotension. She has been prescribed a rate of 0.2 mcg/kg per min, and her notes show her most recent weight was 69.8 kg. The nurses have infusion bags of 20 mg noradrenaline in 480 mL of 5% glucose. At what rate (mL/h) should the infusion pump be set to give the required dose? Give your answer to one decimal place.

22 A 5-year-old child has been prescribed *Gaviscon* suspension 2.5 mL four times a day. *Gaviscon* suspension contains 9.3 mmol Na^+/15 mL. The recommended daily allowance (RDA) of salt for a 5-year-old child is 3 g (equivalent to 1.2 g sodium) per day.
The atomic mass of sodium is 23.
What percentage of this child's recommended daily salt allowance is contained in each dose of Gaviscon suspension? Give your answer to the nearest whole number.

23 Miss K is given an intravenous dose of a drug and her peak serum level is found to be 112 mcg/mL. Six hours later her serum concentration is found to be 0.0035 g/L. What is the elimination half-life ($t_{1/2}$) of the drug in Miss K? You may assume that the distribution is complete and that the elimination is described by a first-order process.

24 You are working for a pharmaceutical company where you are required to calculate the weight of potassium chloride in large quantities of solution before it is prepared. How many grams of potassium chloride are

needed to prepare 3.5 L of a solution containing 16 mmol of potassium ions per 20 mL? Give your answer to the nearest whole number.

[Atomic weight of potassium = 39; atomic weight of chlorine = 35.5.]

25 You have been asked to prepare 0.6 L of a 0.06 g/15 mL solution of a drug for the treatment of magnesium deficiency. You have available, in the dispensary, a vial containing 0.075 g of the drug, which you dissolve in 50 mL of water. How much of this dilute solution (L) will you need to prepare the 0.06 g/15 mL solution? Give your answer to one decimal place.

26 You are working as a practice pharmacist and are helping the practice reduce expenditure on medicines. As a result you are reviewing the use of emollients. Current costs are shown below:

Epaderm	£5.99/500 g
Diprobase	£4.08/500 g

There are 135 patients in the practice cohort who are using *Epaderm*, and you send a letter to each of them asking if they would be willing to switch. The patients are allocated one × 500 g tub per monthly repeat. How much money could be saved over a 12-month period if 110 of the eligible patients agreed to be converted to *Diprobase*? Give your answer to the nearest pound.

27 A consultant dermatologist in your hospital has called to ask if you could mix 125 g of 1.25% (w/w) hydrocortisone with 75 g of 2.5% (w/w) hydrocortisone for one of his patients. What will the concentration (% w/w) of hydrocortisone be in the final mixture? Give your answer to the nearest whole number.

28 A cream commonly used in the local district general hospital is being produced in large quantities by an external lab. You work in the hospital pharmacy department, and have been asked to provide the details of the cream to the lab, so that they can begin large-scale production. The cream contains the following ingredients:

Propylene glycol PhEur 25%
Fractionated coconut oil PhEur 17.5%
Sodium hydroxide PhEur 0.05%
Purified water PhEur 100%.

What is the weight (g) of sodium hydroxide PhEur needed to produce 180 kg of the cream?

29 Mrs D is currently on a heparin infusion to aid in the maintenance of catheter patency. It's 5.30pm and during your ward round you notice her pump is beeping and showing an occlusion, and you alert the nurse who presses the 'stop' button. The junior doctor arrives for his ward round and asks you how much heparin Mrs D has had so far today. The last rate set on the pump was 1.75 mL/h and it has not altered since it was set up at 8am this morning. Her prescription reads 25 000 units in 50 mL sodium chloride 0.9%. How many units of heparin has Mrs D received so far? Give your answer to the nearest whole number.

30 A junior nurse asks for your advice on reconstituting a 2.25 g vial of *Tazocin* (piperacillin/tazobactam 2 g/0.25 g). She is to reconstitute one vial to 10 mL using water for injection, and then add 1 mL of this solution to make up to a total volume of 100 mL with glucose 5%. What is the final concentration (% w/v) of the piperacillin component of this product in the infusion solution? Give your answer to one decimal place.

SECTION C

1   You work for a specials manufacturing company and are required to produce Aromatic Magnesium Carbonate Mixture BP for an order. Calculate the quantities required to produce 350 mL of Aromatic Magnesium Carbonate Mixture BP using the formula:

Light magnesium carbonate	300 mg
Sodium bicarbonate	500 mg
Aromatic cardamom tincture	0.3 mL
Chloroform water, double strength	5 mL
Water to	10 mL

Light magnesium carbonate	mg
Sodium bicarbonate	mg
Aromatic cardamom tincture	mL
Chloroform water, double strength	mL
Water to	mL

2   Mr P is due to commence treatment for chronic myeloid leukaemia. His consultant wants to prescribe the drug busulfan. The dose as stated in the BNF is 60 mcg/kg (max. 4 mg). The patient weighs 10 stones and 2 pounds. What total dose will the consultant need to prescribe? Provide your answer in grams to one decimal place.

(1 lb = 0.45 kg)

3   Mrs F is due to commence treatment for oestrogen-receptor-positive metastatic breast cancer. Her consultant wants to prescribe the drug fulvestrant. The dose as stated in the BNF is 500 mg every 2 weeks for the first three doses, then 500 mg every month. The 500 mg dose should be administered as one 250 mg injection into each buttock. Mrs F's consultant has written up a treatment plan with this drug for 6 months after the first three doses. How many injections in total will Mrs F have received at the end of this treatment plan?

4   Mr K is due to commence treatment for advanced renal cell carcinoma. His consultant wants to prescribe the drug nivolumab as monotherapy. The dose as stated in the BNF is 3 mg/kg every 2 weeks. Mr K weighs

70 kg. Mr K's consultant has written up a treatment plan with this drug for 3 months. What total dose will the consultant need to prescribe? Provide your answer in grams to two decimal places.

5 Mr S is due to commence treatment for advanced renal cell carcinoma. His consultant wants to prescribe the drug nivolumab as monotherapy. The dose as stated in the BNF is 3 mg/kg every 2 weeks. Mr S weighs 65 kg. Each millilitre of concentrate contains 0.1 mmol (2.5 mg) of sodium. The consultant wants to use nivolumab 100 mg/10 mL vials. How much sodium will Mr S receive in his first dose of treatment? Provide your answer in millimoles to two decimal places.

6 Miss F is due to commence treatment for a gastrointestinal stromal tumour. Her consultant wants to prescribe the drug sunitinib. The dose as stated in the BNF is 50 mg once daily for 4 weeks, followed by a 2-week treatment-free period to complete a 6-week cycle. Miss F's consultant has planned for an additional four cycles of treatment, where the dose of sunitinib will be increased by 12.5 mg for the second and third cycles and followed by a further increase of 12.5 mg for the fourth and fifth cycles. What total dose will Miss F receive during her treatment? Provide your answer in grams to one decimal place.

7 You are a medicines optimisation pharmacist and have been asked to estimate the annual cost of an 18-monthly supply of *Epilim* syrup for a 10-year-old child weighing 30 kg. The daily dose regimen is 25 mg/kg. The BNF price for *Epilim* 200 mg/5 mL syrup is £9.78 for a 300-mL bottle. Assume that there are 28 days in 1 month. What is the estimated cost of an 18-month supply of *Epilim* syrup, rounding the total dispensed up to the nearest full bottle? Give your answer in pounds and pence.

8 You are a medicines optimisation pharmacist and have been asked to estimate the annual cost of a 12-month supply of clopidogrel for the prevention of atherothrombotic events after ischaemic stroke. The commissioning group is reviewing the cost of both the generic and the brand product, where the net price of the generic product is £1.83 per 30 tablet-pack and of the branded product is £35.64 per 30 tablet-pack. What is the estimated cost difference of a 12-month supply of clopidogrel for this indication between the generic and the branded product? Assume that there are 30 days in 1 month. Give your answer in pounds and pence.

9   A novel drug therapy is beginning phase 3 trials. It is known that it is principally excreted via the kidneys and is given by intravenous infusion. The dosage recommendations are as follows:

Creatinine clearance (mL/min)	Dosage
>50	5 mg/kg every 12 hours
25–49	2.5 mg/kg every 12 hours
10–24	2.5 mg/kg every 24 hours
<10	1.25 mg/kg every 24 hours

Formula:

$$\text{CrCl (mL/min)} = \frac{1.2\,(140 - \text{age}) \times \text{weight (kg)}}{\text{serum creatinine (micromol/L)}}$$

Mr R is a 60-year-old non-obese male who weighs 75 kg. He is participating in phase 3 trials. His latest serum creatinine level is 138 micromol/L. Using the table above, what is the most appropriate dosage schedule of the drug (mg/kg every hour) for Mr B?

10 The oral dose of a novel therapy to treat small cell carcinoma is 15 mg/m^2 once daily. Calculate the oral dose of this novel therapy, suitable for a 12-year-old child, using the information provided in the table below. Give your answer in milligrams to one decimal place.

Age	Body surface area (m^2)
3	0.23
5	0.45
7	0.79
12	1.17

11 A patient requires treatment with tinzaparin for prophylaxis of deep vein thrombosis prior to orthopaedic surgery at a dose of 50 units/kg. They weigh 11 stones and 5 pounds. How many units of tinzaparin are required to the nearest whole unit?

(1 lb = 0.45 kg)

12 A 2-month-old baby (weighing 5.4 kg) requires prevention of *Haemophilus influenzae* type b (Hib) following close contact with a patient with the infection. The recommended management is rifampicin 10 mg/kg once daily for 4 days. Rifampicin liquid is available as 100 mg/5 mL. How many millilitres of the liquid will be required for the course? Give your answer to one decimal place.

13 Using the following information, how many millimoles (mmol/L) of bicarbonate (as lactate) are there in a 500 mL bag of sodium lactate intravenous infusion? Give your answer to one decimal place.

Ingredient	Amount
Calcium chloride	0.027%
Potassium chloride	0.04%
Sodium chloride	0.6%
Sodium lactate	0.25%
Na^+	131 mmol/L
K^+	5 mmol/L
Ca^{2+}	2 mmol/L
HCO^{3-} (as lactate)	29 mmol/L
Cl^-	111 mmol/L

14 The adult dose of a novel drug therapy to stabilise seizures in West's syndrome, in phase 3 clinical trials, is 150–250 mg daily. Using the information provided in the table below, estimate the daily dose range of the novel drug for a 5-year-old child.

Age (year)	Percentage of adult dose (%)
3	33
5	40
7	50
12	75

15 Mr H has been taking 600 mg of morphine sulfate orally each day. He has been brought to a hospice and is no longer able to swallow. The doctor wants to initiate him on the equivalent dose of diamorphine,

to be given subcutaneously over 12 hours using a syringe driver. The diamorphine infusion that is used contains 2.5 mg/mL. What is the correct infusion rate in mL/h that the syringe driver should be set at? Give your answer to one decimal place.

Oral morphine dose over 24 h (mg)	Parenteral diamorphine dose equivalent over 24 h (mg)
120	40
180	60
240	80
360	120
480	160
600	200

16 A consultant dermatologist requests 500 g of a skin preparation to be prepared by the pharmacy, using the following formula:

Dithranol	2.5%
Salicylic acid	1.5%
White soft paraffin to	100%

Calculate the quantities (g) required to produce 500 g of the preparation.

17 Mr D has been taking 180 mg daily of morphine sulfate via subcutaneous infusion. The doctor wants to initiate him on the equivalent dose of diamorphine, to be given subcutaneously over 12 hours using a syringe driver. The diamorphine infusion that is used contains 2.5 mg/mL. What is the correct infusion rate in mL/h that the syringe driver should be set at? Give your answer to one decimal place.

Subcutaneous infusion of morphine dose over 24 h (mg)	Parenteral diamorphine dose equivalent over 24 h (mg)
120	80
180	120
240	160
300	200

18 Mrs G has been prescribed ferrous sulphate oral drops, 3.2 mL daily. The doctor would like to know how much iron she will receive in this dose. The BNF states that this product contains 25 mg iron/mL. Give your answer in milligrams.

19 Mrs K has been prescribed *Ferrograd* tablets one TDS for 8 weeks. The doctor would like to know how much total iron she will receive over this course. The BNF states that one tablet contains dried ferrous sulphate 325 mg (105 mg elemental iron). Give your answer in grams to one decimal place.

20 Mrs L has been prescribed *Ferrograd Folic* tablets one TDS for 12 weeks. The doctor would like to know how much total iron and folic acid she will receive over this course. The BNF states that one tablet contains dried ferrous sulphate 325 mg (105 mg elemental iron) and folic acid 350 mcg. Give your answer in grams (iron) and milligrams (folic acid) to one decimal place.

21 Mr C is going to be prescribed hydroxycarbamide tablets for the prevention of recurrent painful vaso-occlusive crises associated with sickle cell syndrome. Mr C weighs 72 kg and the doctor would like to write up a treatment plan for:

　　15 mg/kg daily for 12 weeks, then
　　20 mg/daily for 8 weeks.

Hydroxycarbamide is available in 100-mg tablets. How many tablets will the doctor need to prescribe for Mr C for this treatment plan (tablets are not scored)?

22 You have received the following prescription for Mr E:
Anagrelide (as hydrochloride) capsules for the reduction of elevated platelet counts in a patient who is deemed to be at risk of thrombo-haemorrhagic events:

　　500 mcg BD for 1 week, then
　　1.5 mg OD for 1 week, then
　　2 mg OD for 6 weeks.

Anagrelide is available as 500 mcg capsules.
How many capsules are required to be dispensed to fulfil this prescription?

23 Your pharmacy is involved in a Healthy Start Scheme where you are available to provide 'Healthy Start Children's Vitamin Drops' free of charge to under-4s. A 3-year-old child has been referred to the pharmacy to collect the drops. The child's mother would like to know how much vitamin D the child would receive in 1 week from these drops. Provide your answer in micrograms to one decimal place.

> Healthy Start Children's Vitamin Drops, 5 drops contain:
> Vitamin A approx. 700 units
> Vitamin D approx. 300 units (7.5 mcg)
> Ascorbic acid approx. 20 mg

The dose according to the BNF is: child 1 month to 5 years, 5 drops daily.

24 A child who weighs 11 kg is prescribed nitrofurantoin at a dose of 1 mg/kg at night for prophylaxis against recurrent urinary tract infections. How many millilitres of nitrofurantoin suspension 25 mg/5 mL should the child be given per dose? Give your answer to one decimal place.

25 You have received the following prescription for Mrs H:

> Prednisolone 5 mg e/c tablets
> 65 mg OD for 2 weeks then,
> Reduce daily dose by 5 mg per week until course is completed.

How many prednisolone 5mg e/c tablets are required to be dispensed to fulfil this prescription?

26 Mrs S is prescribed 120 mg diamorphine to be administered subcutaneously over 24 hours using a syringe driver. The diamorphine infusion that is used contains 5 mg/mL. What is the correct infusion rate in mL/h that the syringe driver should be set at?

27 A 23-year old man who weighs 65 kg has been brought into the accident and emergency unit as he has been bitten by a poisonous snake. The hospital protocol is to administer the content of one vial (10 mL) of European viper venom antiserum by intravenous infusion over 30 minutes, after diluting it in sodium chloride 0.9% (using 5 mL diluent/kg body weight). What is the correct amount of diluent (mL) required for this patient?

28 A 42-year old woman who weighs 70 kg has been brought into the accident and emergency unit as she has been bitten by a poisonous snake. The hospital protocol is to administer the content of one vial (10 mL) of European viper venom antiserum by intravenous injection over 15 minutes. What is the correct rate in mL/min that the syringe driver should be set at? Give your answer to one decimal place.

29 A 42-year old woman who weighs 63 kg has been admitted to hospital with acute pancreatitis. She has consented to participating in a clinical trial. Drug VB67A is required to be administered to the patient at a dose of 3 mcg/kg per min. The drug infusion to be used contains 250 mg in 50 mL. At what rate should the infusion pump be set? Give your answer in mL/h to one decimal place.

30 A nurse on your ward has calculated the amount of infusion fluid required to make up the aciclovir prescription below and would like you to verify that this is the correct amount. The aciclovir has to be initially reconstituted with water for injection, then added to glucose 5%. Calculate how much infusion fluid should be used to dilute the reconstituted aciclovir to achieve the final concentration prescribed.

Aciclovir		
Dose	Route	Start date
250 mg	IV	TODAY
Signature of doctor	D. Lomas	
Additional comments	Final concentration to be 5 mg/mL	

SECTION D

Oksana Pyzik

1   A 79-year-old man requires oxygen treatment due to his worsening heart failure. He has a 2300 L oxygen cylinder and the prescriber has instructed him to set the flow rate at 2 L/min. If given continuously, how long will the cylinder provide oxygen? Give your answer to the nearest hour.

2   A 50-year-old woman is admitted to hospital due to an overdose of clonazepam. The klonopin blood test showed a plasma concentration of 2.0 mcg/ml. Any level >0.08 mcg/mL is considered toxic and the half-life of clonazepam is 30 hours. How long in hours will it take for the plasma concentration to fall to 0.03125 mcg/mL? Assume that absorption and distribution are complete and elimination is described by a first-order reaction.

3   Vitamin A oral drops are available as an unlicensed special product containing 150 000 units of vitamin A per 30 drops. How much vitamin A (units) is present in 10 drops of this product?

4   Mrs BB's GP would like to gradually withdraw her prednisolone treatment. The GP has issued a prescription with the instructions to take 25 mg daily for 1 week. From week 2 onwards, the daily dose should be reduced by 2.5 mg every 7 days. What is the exact number of prednisolone 2.5mg tablets that will be required for a 42-day supply?

5   A 63-year-old man is taking *Morphgesic* SR 70 mg BD for chronic pain in terminal bowel cancer. He has just been started on *Oramorph* 10 mg/5 mL for breakthrough pain. According to the BNF, the breakthrough dose is one-tenth to one-sixth of the total daily dose. What is the range of *Oramorph* 10 mg/5 mL that this man can safely take? Give your answer in mL to one decimal place.

6   A new drug that aims to reduce the risk of myocardial infarction is entered into a clinical trial. The study included two groups of patients – 2500 patients who took the new drug for 5 years and 2500 patients who received standard therapy. The results of the trial showed that 8% of the patients in the standard therapy group experienced an MI compared with only 2% in the group taking the new drug. Calculate the number needed to treat (NNT) using the formula and data provided in the box below. Give your answer to the nearest whole number.

> **THE KEY FORMULA**
>
> **Calculating a number needed to treat (NNT)**
>
> $$NNT = \frac{1}{(IMPact/TOTact) - (IMPcon/TOTcon)}$$
>
> where:
>
> **IMPact** = number of patients given active treatment achieving the target
>
> **TOTact** = total number of patients given the active treatment
>
> **IMPcon** = number of patients given a control treatment achieving the target
>
> **TOTcon** = total number of patients given the control treatment

7   A 22-year-old man is admitted to hospital for an overdose of verapamil with a toxic plasma concentration of 74 mcg/mL. The drug's half-life is 8.5 hours. Assuming that absorption and distribution are complete and elimination is described by a first-order reaction, calculate in hours how long will it take for the plasma concentration to fall to 2.3125 mcg/mL. Give your answer to the nearest half an hour.

8   Calculate the eGFR (mL/min per 1.73 m^2) of a 17-year-old boy who is suspected of having an acute kidney injury secondary to IV gentamicin. Notes from the ward round indicate that he is 6 feet tall, weighs 72 kg and his current serum creatinine is 415 micromol/L. Give your answer to two decimal places.

   eGFR = 40 × height (cm)/SeCr (micromol/L)
   foot is equivalent to 30 cm

9   A 52-year-old man has been diagnosed with Parkinson's disease. He has been initiated on apomorphine injections in hospital. He has been discharged with a supply of 20 mg/2 mL ampoules and U100 insulin 1-mL syringes with needles. He requires a subcutaneous dose of 1.5 mg. How many units should be drawn up each time when using the syringe?

10 An 80-year-old woman suffers from chronic kidney disease and a current serum creatinine level of 198 micromol/L. Calculate her creatinine clearance (mL/min) using the Cockcroft and Gault formula. Give your answer to the nearest whole number.

Weight: 78 kg
Height: 5′ 8″
Age: 80
Gender: female

$$CrCl = \frac{(140 - age\ [years] \times (Weight\ [kg]) \times F)}{SeCr}$$

where *F* is 1.23 for males and 1.04 for females.

11 Mr C is receiving a diamorphine infusion over 24 hours. He is currently receiving a dose of 150 mg over a 24-hour period using a syringe pump that is calibrated to 36 mm/24 h (note that some syringe pumps are calibrated in mm/h). You increase the rate of infusion to 54 mm/24 h. What dosage (mg) will the patient receive in 24 hours following the increased rate of infusion?

12 A 4-year-old boy weighing 38 kg is travelling to Ghana for a 21-day holiday and has been prescribed *Malarone Paediatric* tablets starting 2 days before entering the endemic area. How many tablets are needed in total?
Use the following extract to answer this question: https://www.evidence.nhs.uk/formulary/bnfc/current/5-infections/54-antiprotozoal-drugs/541-antimalarials/proguanil/proguanil-hydrochloride-with-atovaquone/malarone-paediatric

13 Mr VB has been prescribed hydroxyzine hydrochloride syrup 10 mg/5 mL with the following instructions for use:

Rx: hydroxyzine hydrochloride syrup 10 mg/5 mL
Initially 15 mg ON for 1/52
Then 25 mg ON for 1/52
Then 25 mg BD

Calculate the exact volume (mL) of hydroxyzine hydrochloride syrup 10 mg/5 mL required for a 28-day supply.

14 A 44-year-old woman has been diagnosed with iron-deficiency anaemia. She has been prescribed iron sucrose with her target haemoglobin level being 15 g/dL. You retrieve the following information from her summary care record:

> Weight: 76.5 kg
> Height: 5′ 4″
> Iron: 6.9 micromol/L
> Haemoglobin: 8.8 g/dL
> BP: 130/72 mmHg

Calculate the total dose of iron that this patient should receive over the course of the treatment. Give your answer to the nearest 50 mg.

> Total iron dose (mg) = body weight (kg) × {[target Hb (g/dL) − actual Hb (g/dL)] × 2.4} + X

where X is the milligrams of iron needed to replenish iron stores.

X = 500 mg (or 15 mg/kg in patients weighing <35 kg)

15 A 3-month-old infant weighing 6 kg has been prescribed folic acid at a dose of 500 mcg/kg per day. The folic acid syrup you have in stock contains 62.5 mg of folic acid per 125 mL. What volume (mL) of syrup should be given daily?

16 A 20-year-old man is travelling to Cambodia for 6 weeks and has been prescribed doxycycline 100 mg capsules. The patient is to start the course 2 days before entering Cambodia and continue for 4 weeks after leaving. You do not have 100 mg capsules in stock and so agree to dispense 50 mg capsules instead. How many doxycycline 50 mg capsules will you dispense?

17 A coated tablet has a dry weight coating of 10 mg/tablet. The coating solution is prepared to contain 10% (w/v) of coating material. How long (hours/min) is needed to coat a batch of 1 million tablets at a spray rate of 250 mL/min, given that coating efficiency is 100%?

18 A child weighing 6.6 kg is prescribed a dose of 12 mg/kg per day of ciprofloxacin, to be given by IV infusion in two divided doses. What volume (mL) of ciprofloxacin infusion 2 mg/mL should be given for each dose? Give your answer to the nearest whole number.

19 Calculate the volume (mL) of solution that is required to fulfil the following prescription with an overage of 6 mL to allow for any losses on transfer.

> Rx. Ranitidine 75 mg/5 mL oral solution 15 mg TDS for 7 days

20 A 52-year-old man is in the advanced stages of lung cancer and undergoing palliative care treatment. He is prescribed a diamorphine syringe driver and usually takes oral morphine 180 mg BD to control his pain. The syringe driver contains 15 mL of diamorphine 20 mg/mL. What rate should the syringe driver be set at (in mL/h) so the patient receives the equivalent dose of diamorphine? Give your answer to two decimal places.

Equivalent doses of morphine sulfate and diamorphine hydrochloride given over 24 hours
These equivalences are *approximate only* and should be adjusted according to response

MORPHINE		PARENTERAL DIAMORPHINE
Oral morphine sulfate	Subcutaneous infusion of morphine sulfate	Subcutaneous infusion of diamorphine hydrochloride
over 24 hours	over 24 hours	over 24 hours
30 mg	15 mg	10 mg
60 mg	30 mg	20 mg
90 mg	45 mg	30 mg
120 mg	60 mg	40 mg
180 mg	90 mg	60 mg
240 mg	120 mg	80 mg
360 mg	180 mg	120 mg
480 mg	240 mg	160 mg
600 mg	300 mg	200 mg
780 mg	390 mg	260 mg
960 mg	480 mg	320 mg
1200 mg	600 mg	400 mg

Single best answers

SECTION A

1 C

See BNF, Chapter 1, section 11 under stoma care. Reducing the secretion of acid is the aim in these patients so a PPI, such as lansoprazole, is first-line treatment.

2 E

See BNF, Chapter 2, section 7 under nitrates. Patients require a nitrate free period. Therefore, the modified release preparations should be taken only once daily. This increase in dose may indicate nitrate tolerance and the medicine should be reviewed by the GP.

3 D

Aspirin and clopidogrel are not sufficient to treat and prevent DVT, therefore an anticoagulant is needed. Given the patient's lifestyle it is unlikely he would be able to manage with warfarin. Oral medicines are more acceptable to patients than injections. Thus, rivaroxaban would be the best option.

4 B

See section 7 of the PIL – ensure that button is released and to exhale before putting the inhaler to the mouth. Candidates should be able to determine the technique by understanding it is a DPI rather than a pMDI.

5 E

See BNFC, Chapter 3, section 1 under salbutamol. Up to 10 puffs (1 mg) can be inhaled through the spacer using tidal breathing.

6 E

An understanding of pharmacology is required here. The combination of MAOIs and other agents that increase systemic concentrations of serotonin, such as tramadol, should be avoided due to the risk of serotonin syndrome. Although there is a theoretical risk of increased exposure to opioids in patients taking MOAIs (although see interaction with pethidine), this would not contraindicate their use. For more information on pharmacology see SPCs. For information on serotonin syndrome see UKMi Q&A: https://www.sps.nhs.uk/articles/what-is-serotonin-syndrome-and-which-medicines-cause-it-2.

7 B

See BNF, Chapter 5 antibacterial treatment table. Flucloxacillin is indicated for mild-to-moderate cellulitis. Oral vancomycin is only useful for treatment of *C. difficile* infections. IV vancomycin is a high-risk medicine and is generally used only in hospitals when the patient is penicillin allergic or has a resistant organism. Fusidic acid is generally used only in staphylococcal infections – usually in combination with other agents.

8 D

See SPC, section 4.2. The SPC only contraindicates the use of meropenem when there is history of beta-lactam anaphylaxis or severe hypersensitivity. Vomiting with oral penicillins is not a severe reaction, therefore meropenem can be used in these circumstances. For more information on penicillin allergies candidates are directed to this PJ Article: Penicillin allergy: identification and management (4 September 2015).

9 B

See BNF, Chapter 6 under dapagliflozin and the supporting preamble for SGLT2 inhibitors. Knowledge of pharmacology (see SPCs) is helpful here.

10 E

See BNF, Chapter 6, section 9.1 under supporting information for anti-thyroid drugs and monograph for carbimazole. These symptoms may be a sign of infection secondary to bone marrow suppression.

11 D
> See BNF, Chapter 7, section 6.2 under estradiol. Uterine fibroids do not contraindicate the use of these topical oestrogens, but the patient's fibroids should be monitored in case they increase in size.

12 C
> See BNF, Chapter 8, section 2 for information on common adverse effects of chemotherapy. Patients with lymphoma and leukaemia are at risk of tumour lysis syndrome, which is characterised by electrolyte disturbances secondary to cell lysis. Candidates should be aware of tumour lysis syndrome (characterised the by electrolyte disturbances given) and also have an awareness of the common ranges for blood electrolytes and the symptoms caused when they are deranged http://bestpractice.bmj.com/topics/en-gb/936.

13 D
> See BNF, Chapter 9, section 1. Most patients need to take oral iron for 3 months after their haemoglobin has reached normal levels. If a patient has had parenteral iron they should not take oral iron until 5 days after the last parenteral dose (see cautions for each parenteral formulation).

14 D
> See BNF, Chapter 8, section 2. Only 2.5 mg tablets should be used as per national guidance. See important safety information box that accompanies the methotrexate monograph.
> $15 \div 2.5 = 6$ tablets per dose, therefore $4 \times 6 = 24$ tablets

15 A
> This case is indicative of mild, viral, conjunctivitis that should be managed with simple eye cleansing. None of the products listed are licensed OTC for a child of this age; GP referral is not required initially unless the conjunctivitis is severe or persistent, the child is systemically unwell, there is pain in the eye or there are visual changes.

16 B
> See BNF, Chapter 12, section 2 under chlorhexidine mouth products. If mucosal irritation occurs then the product can be diluted in an

ANSWERS

equal amount of water. The description given is characteristic of mucosal irritation and desquamation.

17 E

See BNF, Appendix 1, table of interactions and MHRA warnings about warfarin interaction with topical miconazole: https://www.gov.uk/drug-safety-update/topical-miconazole-including-oral-gel-reminder-of-potential-for-serious-interactions-with-warfarin.

18 B

See BNF, Chapter 13, section 1 under administration advice for paraffin-containing emollient creams and ointments. This advice will maximise skin hydration and avoid the development of folliculitis.

19 E

See BNF, Chapter 14, section 4 under the indications for each vaccine. Patients who have suffered a severe head injury such as this are at increased risk of pneumococcal infection and therefore should receive the 23-valent pneumococcal vaccine.

20 A

See BNF Chapter 14, section 2 under lidocaine for indication and dose information for lidocaine medicated plasters.

21 D

Section 6.6 of the SPC states that it should be diluted to a concentration not exceeding 10 mg/mL, therefore only D and E are appropriate for administration. However, you need to ensure that the least amount of fluid is given therefore D achieves this. See BNF, Chapter 4, section 2 under phenytoin for supporting information.

22 A

See BNF, Chapter 16, section 1. Candidates should also endeavour to know when the other agents listed here are used in emergency settings.

23 D

See BNF, Appendix 4. Hydrogel dressings should be avoided in heavily exuding or infected wounds.

24 C

See section 4.2 of the SPC for dosing information in renal impairment. Note that many hospitals follow the guidance given in the renal drug database of 1.2 g (1000/200 mg) every 12 hours, when the CrCl is between 10 and 30 mL/min. However, as this question specifically references the SPC, this should be used here (and this information is reflected in the BNF).

25 E

See the continuous subcutaneous infusions information in the palliative care section at the beginning of the BNF. Water for injections should be used to make up the syringe to an appropriate volume because sodium chloride can increase the risk of precipitation.

26 D

As an alpha blocker tamsulosin can cause drops in blood pressure and therefore carries the greatest risk of falls in this list of medicines. Galantamine has a lower associated risk of falls. Warfarin does not precipitate falls but patients taking this should be assessed for bleeding after falls. For more information on reviewing patients who fall, please see NICE CG 161 (falls in older people: assessing risk and prevention) and the British Geriatrics Society (see their medicines and falls in hospital guide).

27 A

Signatures of the overall authorising medic/dentist and pharmacist are required. The PGD must specify what records need to be kept, which could be in the GP, pharmacy or hospital records. See the Human Medicines Regulations 2012 for the full legislation around PGDs, or read this MHRA guidance: https://www.gov .uk/government/publications/patient-group-directions-pgds/patient-group-directions-who-can-use-them#legal-requirements.

28 C

The total effect for bacteriological cure crosses the centre line and the CI traverses 1, therefore there is no significant difference between treatments. However, the total (diamond) for symptomatic cure is clearly in favour of antibiotic 2 and does not touch the centre line.

ANSWERS

29 B
Levodopa can cause nausea, and domperidone is a dopamine antagonist, so it is a useful agent in the treatment of nausea in these patients. Note the issues of using metoclopramide and hyoscine in these patients.

30 D
See BNFC, Chapter 1, section 10. Pancreatin contains enzymes that are denatured in extremes of heat.

SECTION B

1 C

Cross sectional study. Definition of each at http://www.nhs.uk/news/
Pages/Newsglossary.aspx

A - A case series is a descriptive study of a group of people, who
usually receive the same treatment or who have the same disease.
This type of study can describe characteristics or outcomes in a
particular group of people, but cannot determine how they compare
with people who are treated differently or who do not have the
condition.

B – A cohort study identifies a group of people and follows them over
a period of time to see how their exposures affect their outcomes.
This type of study is normally used to look at the effect of suspected
risk factors that cannot be controlled experimentally, e.g. the effect
of smoking on lung cancer.

D – A longitudinal study is one that studies a group of people over
time.

E – A prospective observational study identifies a group of people
and follows them over a period of time to see how their exposures
affect their outcomes. A prospective observational study is normally
used to look at the effect of suspected risk factors that cannot be
controlled experimentally, such as the effect of smoking on lung
cancer.

2 B

See BNF, Chapter 4, section 3.6.

3 C

See MEP 41, p120. Registers should be kept for 2 years from the
date of the last entry.

4 B

See BNF, Appendix 1

Rivaroxaban + clopidogrel are licensed for prevention of
atherothrombotic events after an ACS with elevated biomarkers.
After a TIA, and now AF, monotherapy is sufficient. Refer to NICE
guidance TA256. Caution should be taken with concomitant use of
drugs that increase the risk of bleeding.

ANSWERS

5 C
See GPhC guidance on raising concerns.

6 A
See BNF, Chapter 6, section 8 – Reasons to stop HRT.
A blood pressure reading >160/>95 mmHg is a reason to stop. All other options are correct.

7 B
See BNF, Chapter 4, section 5

>   A   lowest effective dose for *shortest* possible duration
>   B   is the correct answer
>   C   increased risk of serious *cardiac* side-effects
>   D   10 mg up to TDS
>   E   max. dose 10 mg TDS

8 B
Best to spread over 3 days or more, not 2.

9 D
See BNF, Chapter 4, section 2
There are three categories of anti epileptics described in the BNF:

1   Phenytoin is Category 1 – patient should be maintained on the same brand.
2   Clonazepam is Category 2 – whether or not same brand is required is based on clinical judgement.
3   The others listed are in Category 3 – same brand usually not necessary.

10 E
The five stages of behaviour change are:

1   pre-contemplation
2   contemplation
3   planning/preparation
4   action
5   maintenance – then possibly relapse.

11 D
See BNF, Preface – Adverse reactions to drugs.

ANSWERS

12 E
See BNF, Chapter 2, section 3.2

- Unfractionated heparin has a shorter duration of action than LMWH, and therefore its effects can be terminated rapidly by stopping the infusion.
- An LMWH standard prophylactic regimen does not require anticoagulant monitoring.

13 A
Carbamazepine is an enzyme inducer. As a result warfarin is metabolised more rapidly, which means its anticoagulant effect diminishes and the INR falls.

14 C
See https://www.pharmacyregulation.org/spp
The standards need to be met at all times, not only during working hours. This is because the attitudes and behaviours of professionals outside of work can affect the trust and confidence of patients and the public in pharmacy professionals.

15 C
See https://www.gov.uk/government/publications/uk-physical-activity-guidelines

A   Gov.uk has produced guidelines for physical activity for all ages including children <5
B   Being active for at least 1 hour a day is the guideline for 5–18 year olds
C   Is the correct answer – children of pre-school age who are capable of walking unaided should be physically active daily for at least 180 minutes (3 hours), spread throughout the day
D   This is not recommended
E   These guidelines refer to 19–64 year olds

16 D
See MEP 41, p.95 – 'The Veterinary Cascade'. With regard to option D, the medicine must be an EU-licensed veterinary medicine.

ANSWERS

17 A

Refer to MEP, Appendix 11 'GPhC guidance on responding to complaints and concerns'. In the case of a dispensing error, an apology should not be confused with an admission of liability.

18 C

See 'Joint statement from the Chief Executives of statutory regulators of healthcare professionals' on the GPhC website.

19 D

Refer to MEP, Appendix 4 'GPhC guidance on patient confidentiality'.

Get the patient's consent to share the information. However, you do not need to do this if:

- disclosure is required by law
- the disclosure can be justified in the public interest
- to do so is impracticable, would put you or others at risk of serious harm, or would prejudice the purpose of the disclosure.

20 C

See BNF, Appendix 1. Since isotretinoin is a retinoid it is closely related to vitamin A. It is therefore important not to take any supplements containing vitamin A, because this could cause hypervitaminosis A.

21 D

See BNF, Chapter 5, section 2. Lymecycline is a tetracycline that should not be given to breast-feeding women. The other options are appropriate to use if necessary in breast-feeding women.

22 C

See www.rpharms.com/resources/quick-reference-guides/tranexamic-acid-p-medicine

    A   Tranexamic belongs to a group of medicines called antifibrinolytic drugs

    B   Licensed from age 18 to age 45 years

    C   Correct answer

    D   The usual dose for menorrhagia is two 500-mg tablets three times a day for a maximum of 4 days

    E   Side-effects can be resolved by decreasing the dose

23 C

See BNF, Appendix 1. Increased serotoninergic effects when SSRIs given with St John's wort.

24 D

See https://cks.nice.org.uk/threadworm#!topicsummary

> A Threadworms are common, but they usually live for 6 weeks in the body. This does not mean that no treatment is required, because often there is a continuous cycle of eggs hatching
>
> B Mebendazole is licensed for children aged >2 years. See BNFC or BNF, Chapter 5, section 4 under mebendazole
>
> C Washing the child's linen is important as soon as treatment has commenced; however, it is not the most appropriate advice because no treatment was offered
>
> D Correct answer
>
> E Permethrin cream is typically used to treat scabies and crabs, and therefore is not an appropriate treatment

25 C

See BNF, Chapter 4, section 6.

26 B

Refer to SPC of orlistat 120 mg. The other options are fat soluble; vitamins B and C are water soluble. If a multivitamin supplement is recommended, it should be taken at least 2 hours after the administration of orlistat or at bedtime.

27 A

- Patients should tilt their head backwards with nasal preparations.
- Blow your nose before using a nasal spray.
- Buccal tablets should be placed high up along your top gum, under the upper lip either side of your mouth.
- Dry powder inhalers: breathe in strongly for as long as you can.

28 A

See BNF, Chapter 2, section 7.1 and SPC. The effects last 20–30 minutes. They can cause postural hypotension so are best taken sitting down. GTN tablets should be supplied in glass containers, closed with a foil-lined cap and containing no cotton-wool wadding because it is adsorbed by plastic.

29 B
See CKS summary: https://cks.nice.org.uk/fungal-skin-infection-body-and-groin#!scenario

30 D
See BNF, Chapter 5, section 2.5.

31 D
Refer to multi-dose regimens for aminoglycosides. Amikacin works effectively the higher the concentration of the drug is in excess of the MIC of the target organism. The higher the peak, the greater the bactericidal activity, so we want a decent peak of 29, although the trough is too high, so we want to leave the dose the same because it is achieving a good peak; however, we need to reduce the frequency at which we're giving it because the patient is not clearing the drug back to appropriate (trough <10) levels.

32 D
See BNF, Chapter 6, section 3.1.

33 E
See MEP. Invoices do not have to be retained for Schedule 2 CDs.

34 D
See BNF, Preface – Prescribing in renal impairment. 15–29 is severe (stage 4) impairment.

35 B

- Medicines that block dopamine receptors should be avoided in Parkinson's disease. The antiemetics metoclopramide and prochlorperazine should be avoided.
- The antiemetic of choice in Parkinson's disease is domperidone; however, the MHRA advice on risk of cardiac side-effects must be recognised.
- Cyclizine or a 5-HT$_3$ antagonist such as ondansetron would be alternative antiemetic option if domperidone were unsuitable.

36 B

See BNF, Chapter 4, section 3.3. Patients should avoid dietary changes that may increase or decrease Na^+ levels (not K^+). *Hypo*natraemia can predispose patients to lithium toxicity.

37 C

See back of BNF, Medical emergencies in the community. 0.5 mL for ≥ 12 years, 0.15 mL for ≤ 5 years.

38 C

See MEP, Appendix 3.

39 B

Patients should not abruptly stop treatment with valproate, and instead see their prescriber urgently. For further information on dispensing valproate for female patients, see MEP.

40 E

Conjunctivitis is a very common side-effect of taking oral isotretinoin.

For options A–E refer to the MEP on supplying isotretinoin and pregnancy prevention.

Not all women need to be on the PPP: the prescriber may agree that there are compelling reasons to indicate no risk of pregnancy (e.g. hysterectomy). The PPP should be in place during treatment to protect female patients from pregnancy and should continue for at least 1 month after stopping oral isotretinoin. Under the PPP, prescriptions are valid for only 7 days. Prescriptions presented after 14 days should be considered expired. For all patients on isotretinoin, a maximum of 30 days' supply can be given.

ANSWERS

SECTION C

1 E

See SPC, section 4.8, Undesirable effects. SPC states that it is very rare and this corresponds to a frequency of <0.01%.

2 E

See SPC, section 4.4, Special warnings and precautions for use. SPC states that reversible increases in serum lithium concentrations and toxicity have been reported during concomitant administration of lithium with ACE inhibitors.

3 C

See SPC, section 4.8, Undesirable effects. SPC states that cough is common – incidence of all others do not match frequency stated on SPC.

4 D

See SPC, section 4.6, Fertility, pregnancy and lactation. SPC states that lisinopril is not recommended during breast-feeding and lithium is a high risk drug, which should not be used in breast-feeding due to reports of neonates showing signs of lithium toxicity.

5 C

ACE inhibitors are less effective in lowering blood pressure in the black population because of low renin levels in this population.

6 B

See SPC, section 4.8, Undesirable effects. SPC states that it is common to develop this symptom and this corresponds to $\geq 1/100$ and $<1/10$.

7 D

See SPC, section 4.5, Interaction with other medicinal product and other forms of interaction. SPC states that carvedilol may potentiate the effects of other concomitantly administered antihypertensives.

8 A

See SPC, section 4.8, Undesirable effects. SPC states that anaemia is common – incidences of all others does not match frequency stated on SPC.

9 B
See SPC, section 4.8, Undesirable effects. SPC states that cardiac arrest may occur – incidence of all others does not match those stated on SPC.

10 E
See SPC, section 4.2, Posology and method of administration. SPC states that according to pharmacokinetic parameters there is no evidence that dose adjustment is necessary.

11 E
See BNF, Chapter 6, section 3.1 under canagliflozin. BNF states that these are signs of volume depletion – patients are advised to report these symptoms and prescriber should consider interrupting treatment if volume depletion occurs.

12 C
See BNF, Chapter 6, section 4 under alendronic acid. BNF states that these are signs of a severe oesophageal reaction and that patients should be advised to stop taking the medication and to seek medical attention.

13 E
MHRA alert states that tachycardia (explained by patient) is a serious side effect that can result in a fatal outcome. This drug needs to be used with caution in patients with cardiac disease.

14 E
See SPC, section 4.8, Undesirable effects. SPC states that this is very rare.

15 A
See SPC, section 4.9, Overdose. SPC states abdominal pain in overdose section.

16 D
See SPC, section 6.4, Special precautions for storage. SPC states protect from moisture.

ANSWERS

17 C

Nothing of note in SPC.

18 E

See SPC, section 4.8, Undesirable effects. SPC states that this is very rare.

19 E

See SPC, section 4.2, Posology and method of administration. SPC states that it is unimpaired by food.

20 A

See SPC, section 6.3, Shelf life. SPC states that it should be stored at 2–8°C in the refrigerator.

21 E

This is not an excipient in this medication so there is no need to do anything.

22 C

See SPC, section 4.5, Interaction with other medicinal product and other forms of interaction. SPC states that the oral typhoid vaccine is inactivated by antibacterials; no specific timeline given in SPC but, if inactivated, it would be more appropriate to reschedule for when course is complete. You can also refer to the BNF monograph for typhoid vaccine to consolidate your learning further.

23 C

MEP states that, for tablets and capsules, blister strips can be removed from their inert outer packaging, but tablets and capsules should not be de-blistered. Following this advice, the blister packs should not be de-blistered.

24 C

See BNF, Chapter 7, section 3.1. BNF states that this is a reason to stop taking the combined oral contraceptive pill immediately.

25 C

See BNF, Chapter 2, section 12. BNF states that this could be indicative of myalgia.

26 A

See BNF, Appendix 1. BNF states that the others interact with aminophylline (increase aminophylline concentration); amoxicillin does not.

27 A

See BNF, Appendix 1 under ACE inhibitors. BNF states that an enhanced hypotensive effect is observed when alcohol is given with ACE inhibitors.

28 A

See BNF, Appendix 1 under alpha blockers. BNF states that an enhanced hypotensive effect is observed when alcohol is given with alpha blockers.

29 D

See BNF, Appendix 1 under tricylic antidepressants. BNF states that an increased sedative effect is observed when alcohol is given with tricyclic antidepressants.

30 A

See BNF, Appendix 1 under antifungals, azoles. BNF states that ketoconazole increases the plasma concentration of apixaban and apixaban's manufacturer advises avoidance of concomitant use. However, the SPC for ketoconazole cream states that there are no known drug–drug interactions to note – the pharmacokinetic section states that plasma levels are undetectable or negligible.

31 C

RPS support alert signposts to http://www.lrsuntory.com, which states that, according to new amounts of sugar in this drink, patients are advised to consume 10 g carbohydrate, so they will need 110 ml.

32 D

Ulipristal is more appropriate because unprotected sexual intercourse took place within a 120-hour period. BNF states that manufacturer advises avoidance, and SPC states that women should not breast-feed for 1 week after taking ulipristal.

33 A
Levonorgesterol is suitable because unprotected sexual intercourse has taken place within a 72-hour period. BNF states that progestogen-only contraceptives do not affect lactation. SPC states that nursing should be avoided for 8 hours after taking levonorgesterol.

34 B
SPC states that for a fingernail infection it can take around 6 months for the infection to be treated: https://www.medicines.org.uk/emc/medicine/29090. Also look at https://www.rpharms.com/resources/quick-reference-guides/amorolfine-5-w-v-nail-lacquer-p-medicine to consolidate your learning.

35 E
Medication history indicates she may have diabetes. This is a referral criterion for this condition because it predisposes to fungal nail infections and could indicate poor glucose control.

36 E
Levothyroxine interacts with orlistat so patient should be referred to GP as per RPS fact sheet. Also see: https://www.rpharms.com/resources/quick-reference-guides/orlistat-60mg-p-medicine#do.

37 E
See BNF, Appendix 1. This patient is taking an antiepileptic. BNF states that there is a possibility of increased risk of convulsions when orlistat is given with anti-epileptics.

38 E
Licensed indication is from age 18 years and this patient is aged 17 years, so should be referred to his GP.

39 E
Licensing for OTC sale states that referral is required if eye inflammation is associated with a rash on the face or scalp.

40 E
Licensing for OTC sale states that referral is required if eye inflammation is associated with a suspected foreign body in the eye.

SECTION D

1 D
Low body weight <50 kg can increase risk of haemorrhage; however, there is no increased risk of bleeding in a patient who is obese. For further information see Table 1 under Special warnings and precautions for use: https://www.medicines.org.uk/emc/medicine/20760

2 A
Acute pyelonephritis is an infection within the renal pelvis, usually accompanied by infection within the renal parenchyma. The source of the infection is often an ascending infection from the bladder, but haematogenous spread can also occur.

3 C
Malassezia yeast germs from the *Malassezia* species may cause cradle cap. The fungal germ lives in the sebum of human skin and may cause an inflammatory reaction in some babies. It is not a contagious condition.

4 A
See BNF, Chapter 7, section 1.2. Finasteride 1 mg tablets are indicated for use to treat androgenic alopecia in men.

5 E
Folic acid 5 mg is recommended for pregnant women with epilepsy. For non-epileptic women the dose of folic acid for pregnant women is 400 mcg.

6 E
High cholesterol is not contraindicated for the OTC use of sildenafil.

7 E
Withdraw anti-epileptics one at a time if on a multiple regimen.

8 C
Pityriasis versicolor can sometimes be confused with vitiligo because they both cause the skin to become discoloured in patches. However, vitiligo often develops symmetrically on both sides of the body simultaneously, whereas pityriasis versicolor may not develop in a

ANSWERS

simultaneous or symmetrical fashion. The skin affected by pityriasis versicolor is usually slightly scaly or flaky, whereas in vitiligo there is usually no change to the texture of the skin. Vitiligo is more common around the mouth, eyes, fingers, wrists, armpits and groin, whereas pityriasis versicolor tends to develop on the chest, stomach, back and upper arms.

9 C

Oropharyngeal cancer is a disease in which malignant (cancer) cells form in the tissues of the oropharynx. Most oropharyngeal cancers are squamous cell carcinomas. Smoking, heavy alcohol use or being infected with human papillomavirus can increase the risk of oropharyngeal cancer. The number of oropharyngeal cancers linked to HPV infection is increasing.

10 A

Erythema migrans (EM) rash is characteristic to Lyme disease.

11 B

Erythematous rash is not a sign of vitamin B_{12} deficiency. Suspect vitamin B_{12} deficiency if the person reports unexplained neurological symptoms (e.g. paraesthesiae, numbness, cognitive changes or visual disturbances). See CKS NICE guidance.

12 C

Macrocytosis may be caused by vitamin B_{12} deficiency, excessive alcohol intake, liver disease, anti-neoplastic drugs, HIV and certain haematological conditions. See CKS NICE guidance: http://cks.nice.org.uk/anaemia-b12-and-folate-deficiency#!diagnosisadditional.

13 D

There is an increased incidence of myopathy if a statin is given at a high dose, or if it is given with a fibrate (the combination of a statin and gemfibrozil should preferably be avoided).

14 E

Superficial spreading melanoma. Around 7 out of 10, or 70%, of all melanomas in the UK are superficial spreading melanomas. It is most common in people with pale skin and freckles.

15 C

A full blood count including a neutrophil count is important to determine if the sore throat is caused by carbimazole inducing bone marrow suppression and thus agranulocytosis.

16 E

The main symptoms of scabies are intense itching and a rash in areas of the body where the mites have burrowed. The itching sensation is strongest at night when the skin is warm. It may take 4–6 weeks before the itching starts because this is how long it takes for the body to react to mite droppings.

17 B

The pessary should be inserted at night. Treatment during the menstrual period should not be performed due to the risk of the pessary being washed out by the menstrual flow. The SPC also advises not to use tampons, intravaginal douches or other vaginal products while using this product. Avoid washing the vulval area with soaps more than once a day as recommended by CKS: https://cks.nice.org .uk/candida-female-genital#!scenario.

18 C

When starting allopurinol, co-prescribe a low dose of a NSAID such as ibuprofen, naproxen or diclofenac, or low-dose colchicine for at least 1 month to prevent acute attacks of gout. Following an acute attack of gout, start allopurinol 1–2 weeks after the inflammation has settled, as the drug may precipitate further attacks (not 4–6 weeks). A urinary output of not less than 2 L/day must be maintained in all patients receiving allopurinol (not 1 L/day). Check the person's serum uric acid (SUA) level and renal function at 3 months (not 6 months). See: https://cks.nice.org.uk/gout#!prescribinginfosub:13.

19 D

Avoid broad spectrum antibiotics due to increased risk of C. *difficile*, MRSA and resistant UTIs. See NICE Management of infection guidance for primary care for consultation and local adaptation: https: //www.nice.org.uk/guidance/conditions-and-diseases/infections/ antibiotic-use.

ANSWERS

20 E

Rotavirus vaccine protects against rotavirus infection, a common cause of childhood diarrhoea and sickness. The vaccine is given at 8 and 12 weeks of age. Rotavirus liquid vaccines are given by mouth (orally) to young infants.

21 E

He is being treated for BPH (benign prostatic hyperplasia) based on dose 5 mg, which is indicated for BPH and symptoms (increased frequency of urination at night). No dose adjustment is required in elderly people. Alcohol does not have a significant interaction profile but advice would be to drink in moderation. Tadalafil exposure (area under the curve or AUC) in patients with diabetes was approximately 19% lower than the AUC value for healthy individuals, but this difference in exposure does not warrant a dose adjustment. Note that the efficacy of tadalafil at 2.5 mg has not been demonstrated for BPH.

22 D

Nitrates are contraindicated as tadalafil significantly enhances the hypotensive effect of nitrates. Note: even in life threatening situations where the use of a nitrate is deemed medically necessary, at least 48 hours should have elapsed after the last dose of tadalafil before nitrate administration is considered. In such circumstances, nitrates should only be administered under close medical supervision with appropriate haemodynamic monitoring.

23 E

Hypotension (<90/50 mmHg), and **uncontrolled** hypertension are CI for patients taking tadalafil. Tadalafil has vasodilating properties hence it can lower BP, which can be dangerous in patients with low BP, but monitor in patients with hypertension. See: https://www.medicines.org.uk/emc/medicine/11363.

24 E

Tamoxifen may increase the risk of endometrial cancer. It increases the efficacy of warfarin and therefore increases susceptibility to high

INR readings. Timing of tamoxifen will not reduce the hot flushes that are a common side effect. Tamoxifen increases the risk of venous thromboembolism and a swollen leg could suggest a deep vein thrombosis, which requires urgent medical attention in a hospital.

25 C

Opioids reduce peristalsis, increase the anal sphincter tone and promote absorption of water from the large intestine; this leads to hard stools and constipation. Ispaghula husk, a bulk-forming laxative, can cause obstruction and increase the risk of faecal impaction in opioid-induced constipation, especially if fluid intake is inadequate. Constipation from opioid use is best treated with a stimulant laxative, a stool-softening laxative or both if necessary. Adequate fluid intake should be maintained. Source MHRA: http://www.mhra.gov.uk/opioids-learning-module/con143740?use secondary=&showpage=6.

26 E

The flu vaccine is safe during any stage of pregnancy, from the first few weeks up to the expected due date. The vaccine does not carry risks for either the mother or her baby. If she has flu while pregnant, it could mean her baby is born prematurely or has a low birth weight. See: http://www.nhs.uk/Conditions/pregnancy-and-baby/Pages/flu-jab-vaccine-pregnant.aspx.

27 A

According to the US Centers for Disease Control and Prevention (CDC), if a woman is exposed to the Zika virus the couple should wait at least 8 weeks after her symptoms started before trying to get pregnant. If a man is exposed, the couple should wait at least 6 months after his symptoms started or last possible Zika virus exposure before trying to conceive. If a woman and man travel together and both are exposed, the couple should wait at least 6 months after their symptoms started or last possible Zika virus exposure before trying to conceive. See: https://www.cdc.gov/zika/pdfs/TravelCounceling-fs.pdf.

28 E

The levels of lithium are above the normal range. Seizure indicates severe lithium toxicity. Lithium excretion is reduced by ACE

ANSWERS

inhibitors and by thiazides. A loop diuretic is the safest option for patients who require a diuretic.

29 A

Viral conjunctivitis is a common self-limiting condition that is typically caused by the adenovirus. While the eye is red it is highly contagious, and for 10–12 days from the onset of symptoms.

30 B

Apixaban is licensed for the prophylaxis of stroke in patients with non-valvular AF and at least one risk factor such as previous stroke.

31 E

Anacal rectal ointment/suppositories: contains a heparinoid.

Anusol cream/ointment/suppositories: contains astringent(s) and an emollient.

Anodesyn ointment/suppositories: contains a local anaesthetic (lidocaine).

Germoloids cream/ointment/suppositories: contains a local anaesthetic (lidocaine) and astringent(s).

Proctosedyl ointment/suppositories: contains a local anaesthetic (cinchocaine) and a corticosteroid (hydrocortisone).

'There is no evidence that any topical haemorrhoidal preparations is more effective than another. The choice of preparation should therefore be based on the risk of adverse effects and the person's symptoms and preference. Preparations containing mild astringents or lubricants relieve local irritation and are less likely to cause skin sensitization. Preparations containing local anaesthetics may alleviate pain, burning, and itching, but can cause sensitization of the anal skin. Lidocaine is the preferred topical anaesthetic because others, including tetracaine, cinchocaine (dibucaine), and pramocaine (pramoxine), are more irritant. Preparations containing corticosteroids may reduce inflammation and pain, but prolonged use may lead to skin atrophy, contact dermatitis, and skin sensitization.'

https://cks.nice.org.uk/haemorrhoids#!prescribinginfosub:1

32 A
Internal haemorrhoids are graded by degree of prolapse (although these classifications do not always reflect the severity of the symptoms). See: https://cks.nice.org.uk/haemorrhoids#!backgroundsub.

33 B
A target INR of 2.5 is recommended for patients with atrial fibrillation according to the British Society of Haematology.

34 E
Severe cases of hepatocellular injury have been reported with tolcapone. Potentially life-threatening hepatotoxicity, including fulminant hepatitis, is reported rarely, usually in women and during the first 6 months, but late-onset liver injury is also reported. Test liver function before treatment, and monitor every 2 weeks for first year, every 4 weeks for next 6 months and then every 8 weeks thereafter (restart monitoring schedule if dose increased). Discontinue if abnormal liver function tests or symptoms of liver disorder. Do not re-introduce tolcapone once discontinued.

35 A
Prophylactic enoxaparin is contraindicated after an acute stroke (for at least 2 months but varies according to hospital).

36 C
Hyaluronidase should not be administered after extravasation of vesicant drugs such as vincristine (unless it is either specifically indicated or used in the saline flush-out technique). See: https://www.medicinescomplete.com/mc/bnf/current/PHP6749-hyaluronidase.htm.

37 C
Levothyroxine is a narrow therapeutic drug so small increases in dose can cause hyperthyroid side effects such as tremor, tachycardia, weight loss, insomnia and anxiety.

38 E
The MMR vaccine is not suitable for prophylaxis following exposure to mumps or rubella because the antibody response to the mumps and rubella components is too slow for effective prophylaxis. Every

ANSWERS

child should receive TWO doses: the first dose should be given to children age 12–13 months; a second dose is given before starting school at age 3 years and 4 months to 5 years. The MMR vaccine may also be used in the control of outbreaks of measles and should be offered to susceptible children aged >6 months who are contacts of a case, within 3 days of exposure to infection. See: https://www.evidence.nhs.uk/formulary/bnf/current/14-immunological-products-and-vaccines/144-vaccines-and-antisera/measles-mumps-and-rubella-mmr-vaccine.

39 C
Ovulation prediction kits detect the surge of luteinising hormone (LH) that occurs 24–48 hours before ovulation. Sexual intercourse in the 48-hour window after the surge in LH should maximise the chance of fertilisation.

40 C
The child presents with classic signs and symptoms of meningitis. When a non-blanching rash is present, it may appear as a: (1) scanty petechial rash (red or purple, non-blanching macules <2 mm in diameter); (2) purpuric (haemorrhagic) rash (spots >2 mm in diameter) – may be absent in early phases and may initially be blanching or macular in nature. Note that images of petechial, purpuric and meningococcal rashes can be found on the Meningitis Research Foundation website: https://www.meningitis.org/meningitis/check-symptoms. Also see CKS: https://cks.nice.org.uk/meningitis-bacterial-meningitis-and-meningococcal-disease#!scenario.

Extended matching
answers

SECTION A

1 F
See BNF monographs and labelling advice. Rifampicin can colour secretions an orange–red colour. Nitrofurantoin can colour urine a yellow–brown colour. Rifampicin is used in combination with other antibiotics to treat infections of prosthetic implants.

2 E
See BNF, Chapter 5, Section 2.6 under urinary tract infections. Public Health England (PHE) guidance is to use nitrofurantoin first line because of high trimethoprim resistance rates. However, there is an increased risk of treatment failure when using nitrofurantoin in patients with poor renal function due to its pharmacokinetics.

3 D
See BNF and PHE guidance on treatment of C. *difficile* infection. Metronidazole is first line for first episodes of mild to moderate infection.

4 H
BNF information for C. *difficile* infection and vancomycin's monograph state that it should be given orally. The SPC for IV vancomycin and capsules also gives more information about this indication.

5 H
This is a well-known reaction, which can occur if vancomycin is given too quickly. See SPC for IV vancomycin for more information.

6 B

See BNF and NICE guidance on the treatment of pneumonias. Clarithromycin can be used to treat atypical pneumonia and should be added to penicillins for the treatment of severe pneumonia.

7 I

See BNF monograph for metformin, which warns about the risk of lactic acidosis in certain situations, including acute heart failure.

8 A

See BNF entries for diabetic ketoacidosis and under the monograph for soluble human insulin.

9 B

See BNF, Chapter 6, section 3.1 under canagliflozin and other SGLT-2 inhibitors. Their pharmacology explains why they increase the risk of developing UTIs.

10 H

See BNF interactions and Stockley's interactions. Linagliptin does not generally cause hypoglycaemia on its own, but can increase the risk when used with a sulfonylurea, metformin or insulin.

11 A

See national guidelines and GOLD standards for the management of COPD, and the use of inhaled steroids in combination with other medicines.

12 D

See BNF, Chapter 3, section 1 and national guidance on the management of severe acute asthma exacerbations which state that continuous nebulised medicines can be used.

13 A

See BNF, Chapter 3, section 1under inhaled corticosteroids and their risk of causing oral candidiasis.

14 G

See BNF, Chapter 16, section 1 under notes with regard to the symptoms of theophylline overdose.

15 H
See BNF, Chapter 3, section 1 monograph and SPC for tiotropium, which advise use with caution if eGFR is less than 50 mL/min/1.73 m^2.

16 G
See BNF, Chapter 3, section 1 monographs and SPC for theophylline, which discuss serum concentration monitoring.

17 E
See BNFC, Chapter4, section 1 under information about status epilepticus.

18 A
See BNF and Stockley's for the interaction between clarithromycin and the anticonvulsants listed. These are typical effects of increased exposure to carbamazepine.

19 G
See BNF and Stockley's for the interaction between meropenem and sodium valproate. This information is also in the SPC for sodium valproate.

20 G
See information in BNF, Chapter 4, section 2. Valproate is associated with the highest risk of malformations, especially neural tube defects. All patients taking anticonvulsants who wish to become pregnant should discuss their options with their GP or obstetrician.

21 H
See BNF, Chapter 2, section 4 under calcium channel blockers. Rate limiting calcium channel blockers such as verapamil and diltiazem should not be used alongside beta blockers.

22 C
Beta blockers should be used with caution in patients with asthma because they can cause bronchospasm.

23 B
Thiazide diuretics are known to increase the risk of gout and may benefit from a medication review.

ANSWERS

24 G

See BNF, Chapter 1, section 2 under methylnaltrexone bromide. Methylnaltrexone should be tried after other agents have failed. More information on its pharmacology can be found in its SPC.

25 E

See BNF, Chapter 1, section 2 under lactulose, which cautions against use in patients with lactose intolerance. Candidates should be able to narrow down the options based on which medicines are available OTC (i.e. GSL or P).

26 D

Although most laxatives should not be used in obstruction, this patient impaction and atony, which is a strict contraindication for ispaghula husk. See BNF and SPC for more information.

27 A

See BNF, Chapter 1, section 2 under arachis oil. Arachis oil must not be used in patients who are allergic to peanuts or soya.

28 C

See BNF, Chapter 1, section 2 under the preamble regarding faecal softeners. Docusate acts as a wetting agent that enables softening of the stool.

29 H

See BNF, Chapter 8, section 1 under patient and carer advice in the monograph for tacrolimus.

30 E

See BNF, Chapter 8, section 2 under methotrexate. Folic acid should be taken on a different day to methotrexate to prevent side-effects..

31 E

Patients taking amiodarone must be warned about the potential harmful effects of sunlight on the skin.

32 D

To avoid oesophageal irritation, patients taking alendronate should do so with a full class of water and remain upright for 30 minutes.

This should be done at least 30 minutes before other medicines or food.

33 F
Lansoprazole should be taken 30 minutes before food for optimal effect.

34 G
Patients should be told to take their metformin during or just after a meal or food to optimise its effects.

35 C
Metal ions can bind to ciprofloxacin, reducing its efficacy.

36 G
Patients should be advised to take sodium valproate with or just after food to reduce gastrointestinal disturbances.

37 D
Meta analyses are the highest level of evidence because they combine the findings from high quality RCTs.

38 A
This describes an audit, which is simply to gather information on the current working practice and compare it with what is expected.

39 F
This describes a PDSA (Plan–Do–Study–Act) cycle. The four stages are described in the scenario. More information is available on the IHI website: www.ihi.org/resources/Pages/Tools/PlanDoStudyAct Worksheet.aspx

40 I
This describes a route cause analysis. The NHS NRLS website contains some more information on this: http://www.nrls.npsa.nhs.uk/resources/collections/root-cause-analysis/

SECTION B

1 A
See BNF, Chapter 14, section 4.

2 H
See BNF, Chapter 14, section 4.

3 D
See BNF, Chapter 14, section 4.

4 C
See BNF, Chapter 14, section 4.

5 E
See BNF, Chapter 5, section 2.

6 C
See BNF, Chapter 6, section 4. MHRA/CHM Advice: Osteonecrosis of the jaw.

7 A
See BNF, Chapter 4, section 4.2 under Impulse control disorders.

8 F
See BNF, Chapter 1, section 2.2 under Osmotic laxatives.

9 H
See BNF, Chapter 1, section 2.2 under Constipation in pregnancy.

10 E
See BNF, Chapter 5, section 2.

11 G
See BNF, Chapter 5, section 2 under Gastro-intestinal system infections bacterial: a first episode of mild to moderate infection, give metronidazole for 10 to 14 days (if no response, second episode or severe, give vancomycin).

12 B
See BNF, Chapter 5, section 2 under genital system infections, bacterial – the antibacterial therapy recommended is azithromycin as

a single dose or doxycycline for 7 days or, alternatively, erythromycin for 14 days.

13 C
See BNF, Chapter 5, section 2.

14 A
See BNF, Chapter, 2 section 6. Should reduce simvastatin dose to 20 mg.

15 H
See BNF, Chapter 2, section 3.2 under Reports of calciphylaxis; MHRA advice.

16 E
See BNF, Chapter 2, section 4 under Step 3 of drug treatment of hypertension.

17 F
See BNF, Chapter 2, section 4.

18 B
See BNF, Chapter 2, section 4.1. Adjunct in heart failure, dose gradually increased if tolerated.

19 B
See BNF, Chapter 6, section 9.1. Patients should be told to report symptoms and signs suggestive of infection, especially sore throat.

20 G
See BNF, Chapter 6, section 9.1. Patients should be told how to recognise signs of liver disorder and seek prompt medical attention.

21 D
See BNF, Chapter 6, section 3.1.

22 C
See BNF, Chapter 6, section 3.1.

23 F
See BNF, Chapter 3, section 1.

ANSWERS

24 D

See BNF, Chapter 5, section 2.

25 B

See BNF, Appendix 1. Increased risk of AV block and bradycardia when cardiac glycosides given with beta blockers.

26 F

See BNF, Appendix 1. Interactions, antiarrhythmic and antipsychotic, both individually prolong Q–T interval, so together there is an even more pronounced effect.

27 D

See BNF, Chapter 2, section 1. Amiodarone can cause both hyper- and hypothyroidism.

28 H

See BNF, Chapter 4, section 2. Hyponatraemia is listed as a common or very common side effect of sodium valproate.

29 B

See BNF, Chapter 2, section 4. There's an increased risk of severe hyperkalaemia when spironolactone is given with ACE inhibitors. The use of these together should be avoided or used at the lowest possible dose for both drugs.

30 G

See BNF, Chapter 2, sections 1 and 4.

SECTION C

1 B
   See BNF, Chapter 3, section 1 under corticosteroids. BNF states that candidiasis is likely to occur with high-dose corticosteroids.

2 D
   See BNF, Chapter 3, section 1 under selective beta-2 agonists. BNF states that fine tremor is likely to occur with salbutamol.

3 C
   See BNF, Chapter 3, section 1 under antimuscarinic bronchodilators. BNF states that dry mouth is likely to occur with antimuscarinic bronchodilators.

4 A
   See BNF, Chapter 3, section 1 under theophylline. BNF states that arrhythmias are a side effect of theophylline.

5 F
   See BNFC, Chapter 3, section 1 under leukotriene receptor antagonists. BNFC states that hyperkinesia is a side-effect of montelukast in young children.

6 H
   See BNF, Chapter 3, section 1 under phosphodiesterase type 4 inhibitors. BNF states that weight loss is a side effect of roflumilast. This is also listed as common in the SPC.

7 G
   See BNF, Chapter 4, section 4.2 under cabergoline. BNF states that a sudden onset of sleep can occur with dopamine-receptor agonists.

8 C
   See BNF, Chapter 4, section 3.4 under amitriptyline hydrochloride. BNF states that antimuscarinic side effects such as dry mouth can occur with tricyclic antidepressants.

9 G
   See BNF, Appendix 1. BNF states that there is an increased risk of bleeding when SSRIs are given with NSAIDs.

10 H

See BNF, Appendix 1. BNF states that there is an increased risk of ventricular arrhythmias when SSRIs are given with quinine.

11 E

See BNF, Appendix 1. BNF states that there is an increased risk of hypokalaemia when loop diuretics are given with beta-2 sympathomimetics.

12 A

See BNF, Appendix 1. BNF states that there is an increased risk of bradycardia (and AV block and myocardial depression) when diltiazem is given with amiodarone.

13 H

See BNF, Appendix 1. BNF states that hypokalaemia caused by diuretics increases risk of ventricular arrhythmias with amisulpiride.

14 D

See BNF, Appendix 1. BNF states that the effects of sulfonylureas are possibly enhanced by chloramphenicol.

15 B

See BNF, Appendix 1. BNF states that there is an increased risk of hyperkalaemia when aldosterone antagonists are given with ciclosporin.

16 A

See BNF, Appendix 1. BNF states that there is an increased risk of bradycardia when non-cardioselective beta blockers are given with adrenaline. This is in response to a rise in blood pressure caused by the adrenaline – although this rise is to treat the hypertension from anaphylaxis and would not result in a hypertensive crisis.

17 A

See BNF under Prescribing in palliative care. BNF states that, for pain management in palliative care, morphine is first line, but this patient is unable to swallow so tablets are not an option. Oxycodone could be another option but the patient does not tolerate it. Therefore, diamorphine would be an appropriate choice of analgesic.

18 F
    See BNF, Chapter 10, section 4. Given that this woman is trying
    to conceive, paracetamol would be the safest option. In the third
    trimester of pregnancy, NSAIDs are associated with a risk of closure
    of fetal ductus arteriosus *in utero* and possibly persistent pulmonary
    hypertension of the newborn. In addition, the onset of labour may
    be delayed and its duration may be increased.

19 H
    See BNF, Chapter 4. The patient requires a strong opioid to control
    pain. As morphine sulfate is excluded, the most appropriate alterna-
    tive to manage the pain is tramadol. Tramadol also has less additive
    potential.

20 D
    See BNF, Chapter 4, section 6. BNF states that morphine sulfate is
    the opioid of choice for oral treatment of severe pain in palliative
    care.

21 G
    See BNF, Chapter 4, section 6. BNF states that pethidine is used as
    analgesia in labour.

22 C
    See BNF, Chapter 10, section 4. BNF states that ibuprofen is indi-
    cated for pain and fever in children.

23 B
    See BNF, Chapter 10, section 4. BNF states that diclofenac can be
    used for postoperative pain. As patient will be sedated and has had a
    previous reaction to opioids, diclofenac suppositories would be the
    safest alternative from the list provided.

24 H
    See MEP, section 3.2.5, Cough and cold medicines for children. MEP
    states that first-line treatment for children with a cough includes
    warm lemon and honey drinks. Codeine linctus would not be a
    suitable option because the MHRA has issued advice that it should
    not be used in children aged <18 years as risks outweigh benefits.

25 G

See MEP, section 3.2.5, Cough and cold medicines for children. MEP states that first-line treatment for children with nasal congestion includes saline nose.

26 F

See MEP, section 3.2.5, Cough and cold medicines for children. MEP states that phenylephrine is unsuitable for children aged <12 years – this boy is 17 so it would be suitable.

27 H

See MEP, section 3.2.5, Cough and cold medicines for children. Codeine linctus would not be a suitable option as MHRA has issued advice that it should not be used in children aged <18 years as risks outweigh benefits. Therefore the safe alternative from the list is warm lemon and honey.

28 E

Paracetamol liquid would be the safest option and, as the child is asthmatic, ibuprofen would be unsuitable.

29 E

Paracetamol liquid would be the safest option as the use of NSAIDs in children with chickenpox is associated with an increased risk of severe skin and soft tissue infections caused by group A streptococci and *Staphylococcus aureus* – see https://cks.nice.org.uk/chickenpox#!scenariorecommendation:2.

30 E

See BNFC, Chapter 10, section 3. Paracetamol liquid would be the safest option as use of NSAIDs in patients with renal impairment is a listed caution and BNF states that use should be avoided if possible.

SECTION D

1 C

The drug prescribed is liraglutide (*Victoza*), which binds to, and activates, the GLP-1 (glucagon-like peptide-1) receptor to increase insulin secretion, suppress glucagon secretion and slow gastric emptying. *Victoza* is indicated for type 2 diabetes mellitus in combination with metformin, or a sulfonylurea, or both, in patients who have not achieved adequate glycaemic control with these drugs alone or in combination. It is also indicated in patients with type 2 diabetes mellitus in combination with basal insulin or both metformin and pioglitazone, when dual therapy with these drugs fails to achieve adequate glycaemic control. See SPC: https://www.medicines.org.uk/emc/medicine/21986#POSOLOGY.

2 E

Nateglinide (*Starlix*) belongs to the meglitinide drug class. It is indicated for combination therapy with metformin in patients with type 2 diabetes inadequately controlled despite a maximally tolerated dose of metformin alone. The primary therapeutic effect of nateglinide is to reduce mealtime glucose (a contributor to HbA1c). Response may also be monitored with 1- to 2-hour post-meal glucose. See SPC: https://www.medicines.org.uk/emc/medicine/25216#CLINICAL_PRECAUTIONS.

3 B

Canagliflozin (*Invokana*) has MHRA/CHM advice (updated April 2016) warning of increased risk of diabetic ketoacidosis (DKA) with sodium–glucose co-transporter 2 (SGLT2) inhibitors. SGLT2-inhibitor induced DKA is a rare but life threatening complication. In patients where DKA is suspected or diagnosed, treatment with canagliflozin should be discontinued immediately. Before initiating canagliflozin, factors in the patient history that may predispose to ketoacidosis should be considered. Patients who may be at higher risk of DKA include patients with a low beta-cell function reserve (e.g. patients with type 2 diabetes and low C-peptide or latent autoimmune diabetes in adults (LADA) or patients with a history of pancreatitis), patients with conditions that lead to restricted food intake or severe dehydration, patients for whom insulin

ANSWERS

doses are reduced and patients with increased insulin requirements due to acute medical illness, surgery or alcohol abuse. SGLT2 inhibitors should be used with caution in these patients. See SPC: https://www.medicines.org.uk/emc/medicine/28400#CLINICAL_PRECAUTIONS.

4 C

See NICE under General anaesthesia: https://bnf.nice.org.uk/drug/ketamine.html#indicationsAndDoses and SPC http://www.medicines.org.uk/emc/medicine/30569.

5 F

See NICE under General anaesthesia: https://bnf.nice.org.uk/drug/propofol.html#indicationsAndDoses and SPC: http://www.medicines.org.uk/emc/medicine/2275.

6 E

See NICE: https://bnf.nice.org.uk/drug/nitrous-oxide.html#directionsForAdministration.

7 B

See NICE: https://bnf.nice.org.uk/drug/etomidate.html.

8 H

See NICE: https://bnf.nice.org.uk/drug/thiopental-sodium.html#indicationsAndDoses.

9 G

See BNF, Chapter 15 under General anaesthesia and NICE: https://bnf.nice.org.uk/drug/sevoflurane.html.

10 D

See NICE: https://bnf.nice.org.uk/drug/neostigmine.html#indicationsAndDoses.

11 A

See BNF, Chapter 5, section 5.2. Chloroquine is used for the *prophylaxis* (not recommended for treatment) of malaria in areas of the world where the risk of chloroquine-resistant falciparum malaria is still low. It is also used with proguanil when chloroquine-resistant falciparum malaria is present, but this regimen may not give optimal protection. See BNF and specific recommendations by country.

12 B

'Photosensitivity manifested by an exaggerated sunburn reaction has been observed in some individuals taking tetracyclines, including doxycycline. Patients likely to be exposed to direct sunlight or ultraviolet light should be advised that this reaction can occur with tetracycline drugs and treatment should be discontinued at the first evidence of skin erythema.' Source SPC: https://www.medicines.org .uk/emc/medicine/26316#CLINICAL_PRECAUTIONS.

13 C

See SPC: https://www.medicines.org.uk/emc/medicine/1701.

14 D

See NICE: https://bnf.nice.org.uk/treatment-summary/malaria-treatment.html.

15 C

See SPC: https://www.medicines.org.uk/emc/medicine/1701.

16 E

Primidone is a structural analogue of phenobarbital and related to barbiturate-derived anticonvulsants. Primidone is largely converted to phenobarbital and phenylethylmalonamide, and this is probably responsible for its antiepileptic action. A low initial dose of primidone is essential. See SPC under pharmacokinetic properties: http://www.medicines.org.uk/emc/medicine/27349#PHARMACO LOGICAL_PROPS.

17 G

See SPC: http://www.medicines.org.uk/emc/medicine/22416.

18 G

See SPC: http://www.medicines.org.uk/emc/medicine/22416
A side effect of topirimate is kidney stones, which in their medical term are referred to as urinary calculi, and sometimes called renal calculi.

19 A

See SPC: http://www.medicines.org.uk/emc/medicine/32510.

20 C

The patient is suffering from status epilepticus. Note that, although IV diazepam is effective in treating status epilepticus, it also carries a high risk of thrombophlebitis, which is reduced by using an emulsion formulation. Absorption of diazepam from intramuscular injection or from suppositories is too slow for treatment of status epilepticus.

21 F

See BNF, Chapter 4, section 2 under Sodium valproate. See under side effects, further information in NICE and BNF: https://bnf.nice .org.uk/drug/sodium-valproate.html#importantSafetyInformations.

22 F

See NICE and BNF: https://bnf.nice.org.uk/drug/sodium-valproate .html#importantSafetyInformations.

23 F

See NICE and BNF under important safety information: https://bnf .nice.org.uk/drug/sodium-valproate.html#importantSafety Informations.

24 A

See BNF, Chapter 14, section 4 under Cholera vaccine. Cholera vaccine is an oral vaccine.

25 E

See BNF, Chapter 14, section 4.

26 G

See BNF, Chapter 14, section 1.

27 C

See BNF, Chapter 14, section 1.

28 E

C-reactive protein (CRP) is an inflammatory marker and predicts the chance of having cardiovascular problems, at least as well as cholesterol levels. See: https://www.health.harvard.edu/heart-health/c-reactive-protein-test-to-screen-for-heart-disease.

29 D
Crigler–Najjar syndrome is a genetic syndrome where an enzyme needed to help move bilirubin out of the blood and into the liver is missing.

30 G
HbA1c is a form of glycated haemoglobin that is measured primarily to identify the 3 month average of plasma glucose concentration. The test is limited to a 3 month average because the lifespan of a red blood cell is 4 months (120 days).

31 F
Creatinine is produced during the normal breakdown of muscle tissue. The kidneys filter the creatinine from the blood into the urine, which is excreted. Creatinine levels are measured to give an indication of kidney function.

32 H
Raised urea may indicate renal injury or upper GI haemorrhage (haemoglobin broken down by gastric acid into urea).

33 D

34 E

35 C

36 A
See BNF, Chapter 7, section 1. The Scottish Medicines Consortium has advised (September 2003) that *Cerazette* should be restricted for use in women who cannot tolerate oestrogen-containing contraceptives, or in whom such preparations are contraindicated.

37 F
See BNF Chapter 7, section 1.2.

38 H

39 G
See BNF, Chapter 7, Section 1.1.

40 G
See BNF, Chapter 7, section1.1.

Calculations answers

SECTION A

1 12.5 mL
Can use allegation method here:

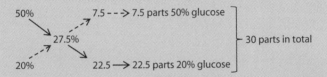

Need to make up 50 mL so 50 mL ÷ 30 parts = 1.6667 mL/part
Therefore: 1.6667 ml/part × 7.5 parts = 12.5003 mL of the 50%
glucose

2 20.9 mL/min
CrCl = [(140 – Age) x Weight × F] ÷ SeCr
Thus, CrCl = [(140 – 81) × 47 × 1.04] ÷ 138 = 20.8980 mL/min

3 3 bottles
Taking 10 mL QDS, thus 40 mL per day, therefore 280 mL over the
course of the week.
This patient can be supplied all bottles because the course length is
not greater than the expiry on the made up suspension.

4 157.5 mcg
250 × 0.63 = 157.5 mcg

5 250 mcg
IBW = 45.5 + (2.3 × 5) = 57 kg

CrCl = [(140 − 71) × 57 × 1.04] ÷ 93 = 43.9819 mL/min
DigCl = (0.053 × 43.9819) + (0.02 × 57) = 3.4710 L/h
Need to rearrange C_{pss} equation to find D. BA becomes 0.63 (due to 63% bioavailable), $t = 24$ hours
Thus: D = [C_{pss} × (DigCl × t)] ÷ BA = [2.0 × (3.4710 × 24)] ÷ 0.63 = 264.4571 mcg
Calculated as top end of the desired serum range. Therefore round down to nearest dose
If use C_{pss} as 1.5 the dose would be 198.3429 mcg, rounded up to 250 mcg
If use C_{pss} as 1.75 (middle range), the dose would be 231.4 mcg, rounded to 250 mcg

6 29.77 g
Total mass need to be made is 30 g (28 + 2 suppositories of 1 g each)
Displacement by morphine = 30 × 12.5 mg ÷ 1.6 = 234.375 mg = 0.234375 g
Therefore, mass of base (*Witepsol*) = 30 g − 0.234375 g = 29.7656 g

7 1.5 m^2
A number to the power of 0.5 is the same as the square root of that number,
i.e. BSA = ([Height (cm) × Weight (kg)] ÷ 3600)$^{0.5}$ = $\sqrt{}$([Height (cm) × Weight (kg)] ÷ 3600)
Therefore, BSA = $\sqrt{}$([123 × 63] ÷ 3600) = $\sqrt{2.1525}$ = 1.4671

8 1263.2 mg
Allegation should be used here:

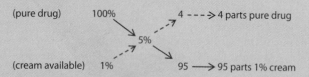

(pure drug)   100%   4 ---> 4 parts pure drug
                      5%
(cream available)   1%   95 ⟶ 95 parts 1% cream

Thus: The 1% cream makes 95 parts of the final product: 30 g ÷ 95 parts = 0.3158 g/part
Therefore: 4 parts × 0.3158 g/part = 1.2632 = 1263.2 mg zinc oxide to add
Can check answer: {[drug in original cream (mg) + mass added (mg)] ÷ [mass of original cream (mg) + mass added (mg)]} × 100
Therefore: ([300 + 1263.2] ÷ [30000 + 1263.2]) × 100 = 5.0001%

9 40 mg

Candidates should know the usual breakthrough pain dose is one-sixth to one-tenth of the total daily morphine equivalent dose. See Prescribing in palliative care information in the BNF.

Total daily dose = 120 + 120 = 240 mg

Thus one-sixth of this = 240 ÷ 6 = 40 mg

10 210 tablets

The SPC states: 'the starting dose is 120 mg twice a day. After 7 days, the dose is increased to the recommended dose of 240 mg twice a day.'

Patient will have 1 week of 1 tablet BD, then 7 weeks (total 8 week supply) of 2 tablets BD.

Thus, amount needed = (1 × 2 × 7) + (2 × 2 × [7 × 7]) = 14 + 196 = 210 tablets

11 2.1 mL

Need 0.5 mmol/kg × 3.78 kg = 1.89 mmol calcium

Calcium chloride dihydrate = $CaCl_2 \cdot 2H_2O$

Thus, need 1.89 mmol of this (1:1 ratio atom to molecule)

Convert molecular mass of $CaCl_2 \cdot 2H_2O$ directly from g/mol to mg/mmol, so 147.01 mg/mmol

Utilise and rearrange molar equation: moles = mass ÷ molar mass → mass = moles × molar mass

Therefore, mass of $CaCl_2 \cdot 2H_2O$ needed is 1.89 mmol × 147.01 mg/mmol = 277.8489 mg

13.4% = 13.4 g in 100 mL, so 134 mg/mL; thus 277.8489 mg ÷ 134 mg/mL = 2.0735 mL

12 630 tablets

Generally easier to draw up a table to calculate the dose

Dose	No. days	No. tabs per day	Total no. tabs
60 mg	14	12	168
55 mg	7	11	77
50 mg	7	10	70
45 mg	7	9	63
40 mg	7	8	56

(*continued*)

ANSWERS

(continued)

Dose	No. days	No. tabs per day	Total no. tabs
35 mg	7	7	49
30 mg	7	6	42
25 mg	7	5	35
20 mg	7	4	28
15 mg	7	3	21
10 mg	7	2	14
5 mg	7	1	7
Total			630

13 150.0 mL/h

Section 4.2 of the SPC states that vancomycin should not be infused faster than 10 mg/min

Concentration in bag = 2000 mg ÷ 500 mL = 4 mg/mL

If fastest rate = 10 mg/min ÷ 4 mg/mL = 2.5 mL/min

Rate per hour = 2.5 mL/min × 60 min = 150 mL/h

Candidates must utilise the decimal and put 150.0 because this is what the infusion pump would read.

14 750 mg

Dose = 15 mg/kg × 49 kg = 735 mg

Tablets are available in 250 mg strength, which are scored and can be halved (125 mg)

Therefore 750 mg should be given (three tablets) because dose range is 15–20 mg/kg OD

15 45.1 kg

Work out target weight: 24 kg/m^2 × (1.56 × 1.56) = 58.4064 kg

Work out how much weight to lose: 103.5 − 58.4064 = 45.0936 kg

16 31 mL

92 mg in solution is equivalent to 100 mg in capsules

Thus 184 mg (92 × 2) of solution is needed per 200 mg dose

30 mg/5 mL = 6 mg/mL

Therefore, 184 mg ÷ 6 mg/mL = 30.6667 mL

17 375 mg
BNF states that 125 mg suppositories equivalent to 100 mg oral
Therefore, 300 mg oral is equivalent to 3 × 125 mg in suppositories
= 375 mg

18 39 capsules
1 capsule on day 1
2 capsules on day 2
Then 3 capsules each day for another 12 days = 36 capsules
Total = 36 + 2 + 1 = 39 capsules

19 50.49 mcg/5 mL
Need to rearrange the equation line to find X
Therefore X (mcg/mL) = $(Y - 0.0470) \div 0.0103$
$X = (0.151 - 0.0470) \div 0.0103 = 10.0971$ mcg/mL
$10.0971 \times 5 = 50.4855$ mcg/5 mL

20 40.32 mmol
Section 4.4 of the SPC states that each 600 mg of product contains
1.68 mmol sodium
Therefore, each 2.4 g dose contains 6.72 mmol sodium (4 × 1.68)
Patient will receive 6 doses per day (24 h ÷ 4-hourly dosing)
Thus, patient will receive 6 × 6.72 mmol = 40.32 mmol sodium

21 75 mcg/h patch
Patient is taking 90 mg BD, which is a total of 180 mg morphine per
day.
BNF states that the closest appropriate patch for this would be a
fentanyl '75' patch.
Candidates should be aware that this represents 75 mcg/h

22 37 tablets
Miss Q is not at risk in Vientiane – see under Laos in the specific
recommendations table.
Miss Q is not at risk in Chiang Mai – see under Thailand in the
specific recommendations table.
However, she is at risk in the forests between these two countries –
see the specific recommendations table. Therefore, she is at risk for
4 weeks.

The recommendations under *length of prophylaxis* state that *Malarone* should be started 1–2 days before entering an endemic area, and finished 1 week after leaving. Asked for the maximum number so need to use 2 days, not 1.

Thus, need to dispense $2 + (4 \times 7) + 7 = 37$ tablets

23 170 ampoules

Will need to use one ampoule to make up each dose of ceftazidime Can use one ampoule for both the pre-dose and the post-dose flush Therefore, two ampoules of 0.9% sodium chloride per dose = 6 ampoules per day (8 hourly = TDS)

Thus $6 \times (4 \times 7) = 168$ ampoules

24 75 mmol

BNF entry for sodium bicarbonate under Prescribing and dispensing information, states that 1.26% gives 12.6 g (150 mmol) sodium/L. This patient is getting 500 mL therefore will receive 75 mmol.

25 8 mL

5 mg dispersed in 10 mL = 0.5 mg/mL Need 4 mg, therefore 8 mL for the morning dose

26 2000 mg

A number to the power of 0.5 is the same as the square root of that number

i.e. BSA = $([\text{Height (cm)} \times \text{Weight (kg)}] \div 3600)^{0.5} = \sqrt{([\text{Height (cm)} \times \text{Weight (kg)}] \div 3600)}$

Therefore, BSA = $\sqrt{([153 \times 61.87] \div 3600)} = \sqrt{2.6295} = 1.6216 \, \text{m}^2$

Thus, dose = $1.6216 \times 1.25 = 2.027 \, \text{g} = 2027 \, \text{mg}$

27 144 tablets

Need 2 tablets per dose $(2 \times 480 = 960)$, which is equivalent to 4 tablets per dosing day $(2 \times \text{BD})$

Only takes these three times a week, therefore will have $4 \times 3 = 12$ tablets per week

Thus, need to supply $12 \times 12 = 144$ tablets for the period

28 19.8 g

See the *N*-acetylcysteine dose and administration tables

For her weight Miss E will receive 49 mL for the first infusion, 17 mL for the second infusion and 33 mL for the third infusion. This gives a total of 99 mL

These tables also state the concentration as 200 mg/mL. Therefore 200 × 99 = 19 800 mg

29 3 packs
He will take 3 tablets on 5 days of the week
He will take 2 tablets on 2 days of the week
Therefore (3 × 5) + (2 × 2) = 19 tablets per week
Thus 19 × 4 = 76 tablets in total
76 ÷ 28 = 2.7143 packs

30 £7645 per 100 patients
Cost per 500 mg vial = £76.90 ÷ 10 = £7.69
Cost per 1 g vial = £153.50 ÷ 10 = £15.35
Current cost per patient = £15.35 × 3 × 5 = £230.25
New cost per patient = £7.69 × 4 × 5 = £153.80
Cost difference per patient = £322.35 − £215.32 = £76.45
Cost difference per 100 patients = 76.45 × 100 = £7645

SECTION B

1 470 tablets
   60 mg (12 tablets) daily for 10 days = 120 tablets
   55 mg (11 tablets) daily for 7 days = 77 tablets
   50 mg (10 tablets) daily for 7 days = 70 tablets
   45 mg (9 tablets) daily for 7 days = 63 tablets
   40 mg (8 tablets) daily for 7 days = 56 tablets
   35 mg (7 tablets) daily for 7 days = 49 tablets
   30 mg (6 tablets) daily for 7 days = 42 tablets
   25 mg (5 tablets) daily for 7 days = 35 tablets
   20 mg (4 tablets) daily for 7 days = 28 tablets
   15 mg (3 tablets) daily for 7 days = 21 tablets
   10 mg (2 tablets) daily for 7 days = 14 tablets
   5 mg (1 tablet) daily for 7 days = 7 tablets
   Total needed = 582; you supply 112 and therefore still owe 470 tablets

2 425 mg/24 h
   320 mg = 36 mm
   X mg = 48 mm
   X mg = (48 mm × 320 mg)/36 mm
   = 426.66 mg = 425 mg to nearest 5 mg

3 57.5 g
   Step 1: 25 supps × 20% = 30 supps total
   Step 2: 30 supps × 125 mg paracetamol = 3750 mg or 3.75 g
   Displacement volume = 1.5, meaning 1.5 g of paracetamol (drug) displaces 1 g of glycerol (base)
   Step 3: If 1.5 g drug displaces 1 g base, 3.75 g drug will displace X g base
   X g = (3.75 g × 1 g)/1.5 g = 2.5 g base (this is the space taken up by all the paracetamol across the whole batch of 30 supps)
   Step 4: Total weight of 30 supps = 30 × 2 g = 60 g total weight
   60 g − 2.5 g base = 57.5 g base required to prepare all suppositories

4 75 mL
   Dose is 0.5 mL/kg × 7 kg = 3.5 mL per dose which is 10.5 mL per day.
   10.5 mL per day is equal to 73.5 mL for 7 days, which is 75 mL to the nearest 5 mL.

5 216 000 units
   60 units × 75 kg three times a week for 4 weeks = 54 000 units
   80 units × 75 kg three times a week for 4 weeks = 72 000 units
   100 units × 75 kg three times a week for 4 weeks = 90 000 units
   Total for 12 weeks = 216 000 units

6 £1783
   800 units:
   Current cost = £29.60 × 25 patients = £740
   Licensed version cost = £3.60 × 25 = £90
   Saving = £740 − £90 = £650
   3200 units:
   Current cost = £58.90 × 13 = £765.70
   Licensed version cost = £13.32 × 13 = £173.16
   Saving = £592.54
   25 000 units:
   Current cost = £112.50 × 5 = £562.50
   Licensed version cost = £4.45 × 5 = £22.25
   Saving = £540.25
   Total = £1782.79; to nearest pound = £1783

7 £116
   200 mg (40 tabs) for 2 days = 80 tablets
   175 mg (35 tabs) for 1 day = 35 tablets
   150 mg (30 tabs) for 1 day = 30 tablets
   125 mg (25 tabs) for 1 day = 25 tablets
   100 mg (20 tabs) for 1 day = 20 tablets
   75 mg (15 tabs) for 1 day = 15 tablets
   50 mg (10 tabs) for 1 day = 10 tablets
   25 mg (5 tabs) for 1 day = 5 tablets
   Total = 220 tablets needed
   Price is £19.50 for 50 tablets, so
   £85.80 for 220 tablets (as 39p per tablet)

ANSWERS

£85.80 × 1.3 (30% markup) = £111.54 + £4.50 dispensing fee = £116.04 = £116 to nearest pound

8 4% w/v
Displacement volume = 0.8 mL/g, so 0.4 mL per 500 mg powder
Final solution will contain 500 mg powder within 12.4 mL of water
The concentration is therefore 500 mg/12.4 mL = 40.32 mg/mL = 4032.25 mg/100 mL = 4.03 g/100 mL = 4% w/v

9 25% w/v
The drug is applied at a concentration of 12.5% (w/v), which has been prepared from a solution that has been diluted 1 in 2.
Therefore, working backwards, if we multiply this by 2 (i.e. 12.5% w/v × 2) this will give us the concentration of the intermediate solution of 25% w/v.
The 48% concentrate strength isn't needed for this calculation.

10 0.01 kg
1 in 15 dilution produces 1 in 6000
Therefore the original concentrate is 15 times stronger, i.e. 1 in 400 (6000/15)
1 in 400 = 1 g in 400 mL = X g in 4325 mL
X g = (1 g × 4325 mL)/400 mL = 10.8125 g = 0.0108 kg = 0.01 kg

11 460 000 units
Two batches of 20 plus extra 15% = (20 × 2) × 1.15 = 46 amps
Each ampoule = 2 mL. Therefore 10 000 units per ampoule
10 000 units × 46 amps = 460 000 units

12 121.5 g
30 supps + 20% extra = 36 supps in total
36 supps × 100 mg tramadol = 3600 mg or 3.6 g of active ingredient
Displacement volume = 0.8, meaning 0.8 g of tramadol will displace 1 g of theobroma oil (the base)
If 0.8 g displaces 1 g, 3.6 g will displace X g
X g = (3.6 g × 1 g)/0.8 g = 4.5 g of base displaced across the whole batch
Total weight of supps = 36 supps × 3.5g = 126 g
126 g − 4.5 g = 121.5 g base

13 72 tablets

One 30 mg tablet is needed for every 12.5 mL of mixture
We need 450 mL of mixture, which is 36 times the recipe (450 mL/12.5 mL)
We therefore need 36 tablets of the 30 mg strength, and so will need double the number of 15 mg tablets, i.e. 72 tablets
Double check: 36 tablets × 30 mg = 1080 mg, and 72 tablets × 15 mg = 1080 mg

14 £1707

Seretide:
The difference in cost between the 250 and the 125 = £59.48 – £35.00 = £24.48
For 12 patients the savings would be £24.48 × 12 patients = £293.76
For 4 months this would be £293.76 × 4 = £1175.04
Symbicort:
The 400/12 inhalers last only for 1 month, whereas the 200/6 inhalers would last for 2 months, halving the costs. This means that each patient switched would save £19.
For 7 patients that would save £19 × 7 = 133
For 4 months this would be £133 × 4 = £532
Total savings = £532 + £1175 = £1707

15 67 days

Spray contains 140 doses, with 50 mcg/dose
2 sprays (100 mcg) OD for 3 days = 6 sprays × 2 nostrils = 12 sprays, therefore 128 doses left in the bottle
Then 1 spray daily (50 mcg) to both nostrils = 2 sprays daily, divided by 128 doses left = 64 days
Total = 64 + 3 = 67 days

16 1.6 mL

Displacement volume = 0.05 mL per 250 mg, therefore in 1000 mg the volume displaced is 0.05 mL × 4 = 0.2 mL
1.75 mL − 0.2 mL = 1.55 mL = 1.6 mL to one decimal place

17 0.12 mcg/mL

How many hours are in each half-life ($t_{1/2}$ = 840 minutes) = 14 hours
5 days and 20 hours = 140 hours

Therefore:

0 hours	126 mcg/mL
14 hours	63 mcg/mL
28 hours	31.5 mcg/mL
42 hours	15.75 mcg/mL
56 hours	7.875 mcg/mL
70 hours	3.9375 mcg/mL
84 hours	1.9687 mcg/mL
98 hours	0.98 mcg/mL
112 hours	0.49 mcg/mL
126 hours	0.245 mcg/mL
140 hours	0.1225 mcg/mL

$= 0.12$ mcg/mL to two decimal places

18 445 mL
   Loading dose is 3.5 mL/kg = 3.5 mL $\times$ 81 kg = 283.5 mL
   283.5 mL (V_1) of 40% (C_1) ethanol required, but only have 25.5% (C_2) gin. V_2 is missing.
   283.5mL $\times$ 40% = 25.5% $\times$ V_2
   $V_2 = 444.705$ mL = 445 mL to the nearest whole number

19 90 mg
   Dose is 7 FTUs per dose
   Applying BD for 14 days = 14 FTUs daily $\times$ 14 days = 196 FTUs
   2 FTUs = 1 g, therefore 196 FTUs = 98 g
   Cream is 0.1% = 0.1 g in 100 g cream, X g in 98 g
   X g = 0.098 g = 98 mg

20 16 tablets
   Final concentration is 0.005%, which is a 1 in 25 diluted solution
   Strength to supply to the patient is 25 $\times$ stronger, i.e. 0.125%. We need to prepare 5 L of a 0.125% solution
   0.125% = 0.125 g in 100 mL = 1.25 g in 1000 mL = 6.25 g in 5 L
   Each tablet is 400 mg so 15.625 tablets needed, rounded up to 16 tablets

21 20.1 mL/h
Patient needs 0.2 mcg × 69.8 kg = 13.96 mcg/min = 837.6 mcg/h
Infusion bag contains 20 000 mcg/480 mL, therefore 837.6 mcg in 20.102 mL
Rate = 20.1 mL/h

22 3%
Each dose is 2.5mL
Gaviscon contains 9.3 mmol Na$^+$/15 mL, therefore 1.55 mmol Na$^+$ in a 2.5 mL dose
Mass = M_r × moles = 23 × 1.55 mmol = 35.65 mg
35.65 mg/1200 mg = 0.0297 × 100 = 3% to the nearest whole number

23 72 minutes
112 mcg/mL; after 6 hours this reduced to 0.0035 g/L
The first step is to convert both numbers into the same units
0.0035 g/L = 3.5 mg/L = 3500 mcg/L = 3.5 mcg/mL
112 – $t_{1/2}$ – 56 – $t_{1/2}$ – 28 – $t_{1/2}$ – 14 – $t_{1/2}$ – 7 – $t_{1/2}$ – 3.5
Five half-lives in 6 hours so one half-life is 72 minutes

24 209 g
1 mole of potassium chloride weighs 74.5 g (39 + 35.5)
1 mmol = 74.5 mg (divide both sides by 1000)
The solution to be prepared contains 16 mmol potassium ions in 20 mL = 8 mmol in 10 mL
= 2800 mmol in 3500 mL (8 mmol × 350)
Mass (g) = M_r × moles = 74.5 mg × 2.8 mol = 208.6 g

25 1.6 L
The required strength is 0.06 g in 15 mL = 60 mg in 15 mL
In 0.6 L (600 mL) you will have (60 mg × 600 mL)/15 mL = 2400 mg
The solution that you have prepared contains 0.075 g in 50 mL (75 mg in 50 mL) = 1.5 mg/mL, therefore 2400 mg in X mL
X mL = (2400 mg × 1 mL)/1.5 mg = 1600 mL = 1.6 L

26 £2521
Epaderm 110 patients × £5.99 = £658.90 for 1 month; × 12 months = £7906.80

Diprobase 110 patients × £4.08 = £448.80 for 1 month; × 12 months = £5385.60
£7906.80 − £5385.60 = £2521.20 = £2521

27 **2% w/w**
1.25% = 1.25 g in 100 g, therefore in 125 g there will be:
(1.25 g × 125 g)/100 g = 1.5625 g
2.5% = 2.5 g in 100 g, therefore in 75 g there will be:
(2.5 g × 75 g)/100 g = 1.875 g
Therefore the final mixture will be 200 g and contain 34375 g hydrocortisone
The percentage strength is (3.4375 g /200 g) × 100% = 1.7187%, rounded up to 2% w/w

28 **90 g**
0.05% of the overall cream is sodium hydroxide
Therefore 0.0005 × 180000 g = 90 g
Alternative working:
0.05% = 0.05 g in 100 g, therefore X g in 180 000 g
X g = 0.05 g/(100 g × 180000 g) = 90 g

29 **8313 units**
8am to 5.30pm = 9.5 hours
Rate = 1.75 mL/h, therefore = 9.5 h × 1.75 mL = 16.625 mL
Heparin = 25 000 units in 50 mL or X units in 16.625 mL
X units = (16.625 mL × 25 000 units)/50mL = 8312.5 units = 8313 units to nearest whole number

30 **0.2%**
2.25 g vial is to be reconstituted to 10mL
This will contain 2,000 mg of piperacillin in 10mL
This is equal to 200 mg in 1mL
We have then to add 1mL (200 mg) and make up to final volume of 100 mL
We will therefore have 200 mg in 100 mL = 0.2% w/v

SECTION C

1 Multiply everything by 35:

Light magnesium carbonate	10 500 mg
Sodium bicarbonate	17 500 mg
Aromatic cardamom tincture	10.5 mL
Chloroform water, double strength	175 mL
Water to	350 mL

2 3.8 g
   10 stones + 2 lb = (14 × 10) + 2 = 142 lb
   So 142 × 0.45 = 63.9 kg
   60 × 63.9 = 3834 mcg
   3834/1000 = 3.384 g = 3.8 g to 1 decimal place

3 18 injections
   500 mg every 2 weeks for the first three doses = 2 injections × 3 = 6 injections
   Then 500 mg for 6 months = 2 injections × 6 = 12
   6 + 12 = 18 injections in total

4 1.26 g
   3 mg/kg every 2 weeks for 3 months = 3 mg/kg for 6 treatments
   3 × 70 = 210 mg per treatment = 210 mg × 6 = 1 260 mg = 1.26 g

5 1.95 mmol
   3 mg/kg for the first dose = 3 mg × 65 = 195 mg
   100 mg/10 mL = 10 mg/mL
   So 195/10 = 19.5 mL required
   19.5 × 0.1 = 1.95 mmol of sodium

6 9.1 g
   First cycle: 50 mg OD for 28 days = 50 × 28 = 1400 mg
   Second cycle: 62.5 mg OD for 28 days = 62.5 × 28 = 1750 mg
   Third cycle: 62.5 mg OD for 28 days = 62.5 × 28 = 1750 mg
   Fourth cycle: 75 mg OD for 28 days = 75 × 28 = 2100 mg
   Fifth cycle: 75 mg OD for 28 days = 75 × 28 = 2100 mg
   Total = 9100 mg = 9.1 g

ANSWERS

7 £312.96
   25 mg × 30 = 750 mg daily
   750 × 504 = 378 000 mg for 18 months
   200 mg in 5 mL, therefore 378 000 mg in 9450 mL
   9450 ÷ 300 = 31.5 bottles, therefore 32 bottles
   £9.78 × 32 = £312.96

8 £405.72
   Generic: £1.83 × 12 = £21.96
   Branded: £35.64 × 12 = £427.68
   Difference: £427.68 − £21.96 = £405.72

9 5 mg/kg every 12 hours
   1.2(140 − 60) × 75
   = [1.2(80) × 75]/138
   = 52.2 mL/min
   Therefore choose 5 mg/kg every 12 hours

10 17.6 mg
   15 mg for 1 m^2 so X mg for 1.17 m^2
   X = 17.55 mg = 17.6 mg to 1 decimal place

11 3578 units
   11 stone + 5 lb = 159 lb
   Convert into kg: 159 × 0.45 = 71.55 kg
   Dose: 50 units/kg
   50 × 71.55 = 3577.5 units = 3578 units

12 10.8 mL
   Dose is 10 mg/kg OD for 4 days
   So, 10 × 5.4 × 1 × 4 = 216 mg
   Liquid is 100 mg in 5 mL (20 mg in 1 mL), so 216 mg in X mL
   X = 216/20 = 10.8 mL

13 14.5 mmol/L
   29/2 = 14.5 mmol/L

14 60–100 mg
   0.40 × 150 = 60 mg and 0.40 × 250 = 100 mg
   So daily dose range is 60–100 mg

15 3.3 mL/h
Using table equivalent dose is 200 mg over 24 h, which is 100 mg over 12 h
100 mg over 12 h = 8.33333333 mg/h
Product contains 2.5 mg/mL, so 8.333333333 mg in X mL
X mL = 8.333333333 mg × 1 mL/2.5
X mL = 3.333333333 mL/h = 3.3 mL/h

16 Multiply everything by 5:
Dithranol: 2.5 g in 100 g = 2.5 × 5 = 12.5 g
Salicylic acid: 1.5 g in 100 g = 1.5 × 5 = 7.5 g
White soft paraffin: 96 g in 100 g = 96 × 5 = 480 g

17 2 mL/h
Using table equivalent dose is 120 mg over 24 h, which is 60 mg over 12 h.
60 mg over 12 h = 5 mg/h
Product contains 2.5 mg/mL, therefore 5 mg in X mL
X mL = (5 × 1 mL)/2.5
X mL = 2 mL/h

18 80 mg
25 mg/mL
3.2 × 25 = 80 mg

19 17.6 g
1 × 3 × 56 = 168 tablets
168 × 105 = 17 640 mg = 17.64 g = 17.6 g to 1 decimal place

20 88.2 mg
1 × 3 × 84 = 252 tablets
252 × 105 = 26 460 mg of iron = 26.46 g of iron = 26.5 g of iron to 1 decimal place
252 × 350 = 88 200 mcg folic acid = 88.2 mg folic acid

21 1708 tablets
First 12 weeks: 15 × 72 = 1080 mg/100 = 10.8 tablets = 11 tablets per day
11 × 7 × 12 = 924 tablets for the first 12 weeks
Then for the next 8 weeks: 20 × 72 = 1440 mg/100 = 14.4 tablets = 14 tablets per day

ANSWERS

$14 \times 7 \times 8 = 784$ tablets for the next 8 weeks

Total number of tablets to prescribe $= 924 + 784 = 1708$ tablets

22 203 capsules

500 mcg (1 capsule) $= 1 \times 2 \times 7 = 14$ capsules

1500 mcg (3 capsules) $= 3 \times 1 \times 7 = 21$ capsules

2000 mcg (4 capsules) $= 4 \times 7 \times 6 = 168$ capsules

Total number of capsules $= 14 + 21 + 168 = 203$ capsules

23 52.5 mcg

Vitamin D, 5 drops contains 7.5 mcg

$7.5 \times 7 = 52.5$ mcg for 7 days

24 2.2 mL

1 mg/kg $= 1 \times 11 = 11$ mg per night

25 mg/5 mL $= 5$ mg/1 mL

11 mg in X mL

$11/5 = 2.2$ mL

25 728 tablets

65 mg daily for 14 days $= 13 \times 1 \times 14 = 182$ tablets

60 mg daily for 7 days $= 12 \times 1 \times 7 = 84$ tablets

55 mg daily for 7 days $= 11 \times 1 \times 7 = 77$ tablets

50 mg daily for 7 days $= 10 \times 1 \times 7 = 70$ tablets

45 mg daily for 7 days $= 9 \times 1 \times 7 = 63$ tablets

40 mg daily for 7 days $= 8 \times 1 \times 7 = 56$ tablets

35 mg daily for 7 days $= 7 \times 1 \times 7 = 49$ tablets

30 mg daily for 7 days $= 6 \times 1 \times 7 = 42$ tablets

25 mg daily for 7 days $= 5 \times 1 \times 7 = 35$ tablets

20 mg daily for 7 days $= 4 \times 1 \times 7 = 28$ tablets

15 mg daily for 7 days $= 3 \times 1 \times 7 = 21$ tablets

10 mg daily for 7 days $= 2 \times 1 \times 7 = 14$ tablets

5 mg daily for 7 days $= 1 \times 1 \times 7 = 7$ tablets

Total of all tablets $= 728$ tablets

26 1 mL/h

$120/5 = 24$ mL

So 120 mg is contained in 24 mL

Over 24 hours,

$24/24 = 1$ mL/h

27 325 mL
    5 mL/kg
    5 × 65 = 325 mL

28 0.7 mL/min
    10 mL over 15 min
    10 mL/15 min
    0.6666666667 mL/min = 0.7 mL/min

29 2.3 mL/h
    Dose is 3 mcg/kg per min = 3 × 63 = 189 mcg/min
    189 × 60 = 11 340 mcg/h = 11.34 mg/h
    Infusion contains 250 mg/50 mL which is 5 mg/1 mL
    11.34/5 = 2.268 mL = 2.3 mL/h to 1 decimal place

30 50 mL
    250 mg drug needs to administered
    Final concentration must be 5 mg/mL, 250/5 = 50 mL

SECTION D

1 19 hours
   V = 2300 L
   2 L = 1 min
   2300 L = X min
   X = 2300 L/2 = 1150 min = 19.166 or 19 hours

2 180 hours
   $t_{1/2}$ = 30 hours
   0 hours = 2.0 mcg/mL
   30 hours = 1.0 mcg/mL
   60 hours = 0.5 mcg/mL
   90 hours = 0.25 mcg/mL
   120 hours = 0.125 mcg/mL
   150 hours = 0.0625 mcg/mL
   180 hours = 0.03125 mcg/mL

3 50 000 units
   150 000 units = 30 drops
   X units = 10 drops
   X = 1 500 000/30 = 50 000 units

4 315 tablets

10 tablets	7 days	70
9 tablets	7 days	63
8 tablets	7 days	56
7 tablets	7 days	49
6 tablets	7 days	42
5 tablets	7 days	35
		= 315 tablets

5 7 mL to 11.5 mL
   One-tenth to one-sixth of total daily dose (140 mg):
   14 mg to 23 mg every 2–4 hours
   7 mL to 11.5 mL every 2–4 hours PRN

6 17
1/[(200/2500) − (50/2500)]
= 1/(0.08 − 0.02) = 16.6 = 17

7 42.5 hours

Hours	Plasma concentration (mcg/mL)
0	74
8.5	37
17	18.5
25.5	9.25
34	4.625
42.5	2.3125

At 42.5 hours the plasma concentration will reach 2.3125 mcg/mL

8 17.35 mL/min per 1.73 m^2
Using the equation provided and knowing that 1 foot is equivalent to 30 cm:
(40 × 180 cm)/415 = 7200/415 =17.349
Rounding to two decimal places = 17.35 mL/min per 1.73 m^2

9 15 units
Apomorphine injection = 20 mg/2 mL
Dose = 1.5 mg → (1.5 mg/20) × 2 mL = 0.15 mL
Each syringe can hold 100 units/1 mL
i.e. 10 units/0.1 mL and 15 units in 0.15 mL

10 25 mL/min
= [(140 − 80 years) × 78 kg × 1.04]/198
= 24.58 mL/min
= 25 mL/min

11 225 mg
150 mg @ 36 mm/24 h increased to 54 mm/24 h = (150 mg × 54 mm)/
36 mm = 225 mg

12 90 tablets
From the extract: prophylaxis of malaria started 1–2 days before entering endemic area and continued for 1 week after leaving.
By mouth:
Child body weight 5–8 kg ½ tablet once daily
Child body weight 8–10 kg ¾ tablet once daily
Child body weight 10–20 kg 1 tablet once daily
Child body weight 20–30 kg 2 tablets once daily
Child body weight 30–40 kg 3 tablets once daily
Child body weight >40 kg use *Malarone* ('standard') tablets
$2 \times 3 = 6$
$21 \times 3 = 63$
$7 \times 3 = 21$
$= 90$ tablets

13 49 mL
The syrup is 10 mg/5 mL
Week 1: 15 mg ON → 7.5 mL × 7 = 52.5 mL
Week 2: 25 mg ON → 12.5 mL × 7 = 87.5 mL
Weeks 3–4: 25 mg BD → 12.5 mL × 2 × 14 = 350 mL
Total = 490 mL

14 1650 mg
Iron dose = 76.5 kg × {[15 – 8.8] × 2.4} + 500 mg
= 76.5 × 14.88 + 500
= 1638.32 mg
= 1650 mg

15 6 mL
500 mcg × 6 kg = 3000 mcg = 3 mg
1 mg = 1000 mcg
62.5 mg/125 mL
3 mg/X mL
$X = (125 \times 3)/62.5 = 6$ mL

16 144 capsules
$2 \times 2 = 4$ capsules
$6 \times 7 = 42$ days x 2 = 84 capsules
$4 \times 7 = 28$ days x 2 = 56 capsules
$4 + 84 + 56 = 144$ capsules

17 6 hours 40 minutes
10 g in 100 mL
25 g in 250 mL
25 g/min
10 000 g/25 = 400 minutes

18 20 mL
12 mg × 6.6 kg = 79.2 mg per day
V = 2 mg/1 mL
79.2/X mL
X = 39.6 mL in two doses = 19.8 mL = 20 mL

19 27 mL
1 mL TDS = 3 mL/day
(3 × 7) + 6 = 27 mL

20 0.25 mL/h
Total morphine dose = 180 × 2 = 360 mg daily
According to table, equivalent to 120 mg diamorphine:
120 mg/24 h = 5 mg every hour
20 mg in 1 mL
5 mg in X mL
X = 0.25 mL required every hour

Index